# Ruck Fit

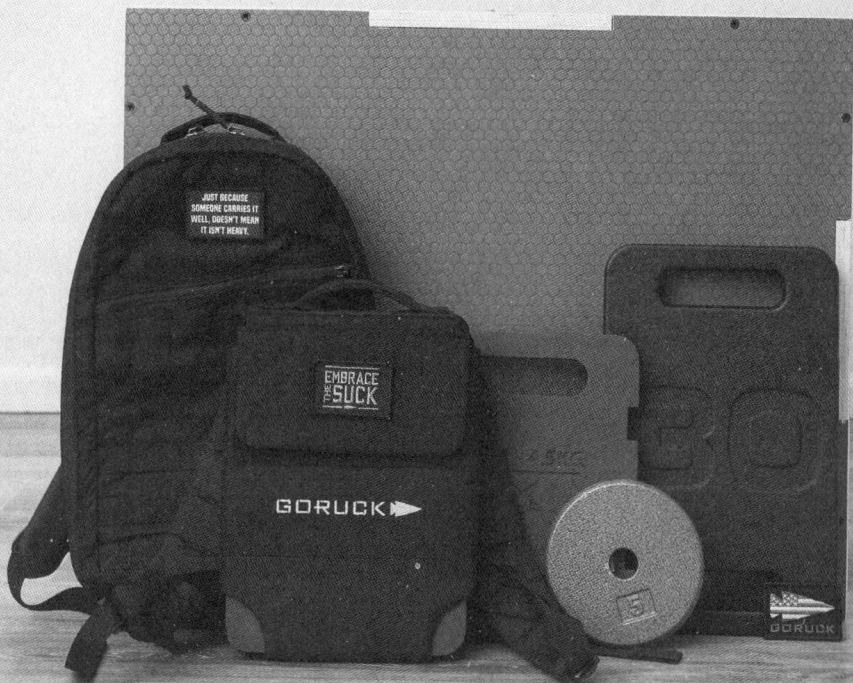

# Ruck Fit

## BUILD STRENGTH AND ENDURANCE BY WALKING WITH WEIGHT

### Kayla Girgen, CPT, RD, LD

Photography by

ERIKA HANSEN

**Countryman Press**

*An Imprint of W. W. Norton & Company*
*Independent Publishers Since 1923*

This book is a general information resource. It is not a substitute for individualized professional medical or physiological care, diagnosis, or treatment. Consult your healthcare provider before starting any new fitness program. Please also note the warnings throughout this book about when you should consult your physician, and follow the instructions for each exercise carefully, since even stretching can cause injuries if performed incorrectly. Individual products recommended by the author are her personal favorites. You need to do your own research to determine which products are right for you.

The names and identifying details of people mentioned in this book have been changed. Any URLs shared in this book refer to websites that existed as of press time. The publisher is not responsible for, and should not be deemed an endorsement or recommendation of, any website other than its own or any content that it did not create. The author, also, is not responsible for any third-party material.

Manufacturing by Versa Press
Book design by Chrissy Kurpeski
Production manager: Devon Zahn

Countryman Press
www.countrymanpress.com

An imprint of W. W. Norton & Company, Inc.
500 Fifth Avenue, New York, NY 10110
www.wwnorton.com

Authorized EU representative: EAS, Mustamäe tee 50, 10621 Tallinn, Estonia

978-1-324-11152-8 (Paperback)

1 2 3 4 5 6 7 8 9 0

To my fellow ruckers—past, present, and future:
May you bear weight on your shoulders, not in your heart.
Carry what matters. Let go of what doesn't.

# Author's Note

This book guides you through the fundamentals of rucking. You don't need to be an athlete to start, but there are two important precautions to consider.

First, consult your physician before beginning, especially if you have any underlying health conditions. Individuals who are pregnant, recovering from surgery, or managing cardiovascular, respiratory, or orthopedic conditions should seek medical clearance before attempting rucking or any of the exercises described in this book.

Second, pay attention to any discomfort or pain. Minor aches can turn into serious issues if ignored. If you experience persistent pain during or after rucking, consult your doctor promptly. Your health and safety come first—listen to your body!

# Contents

# Introduction

If you're struggling mentally,
throw a ruck on your back and just go.

—MATT PECH,
FOUNDER OF RUCK FOR VETERANS

Rucking is a low-impact yet high-reward form of exercise, making it appealing for all ages and fitness levels. Even well-known personalities have embraced it. Several days per week, *Dirty Jobs* host Mike Rowe challenges himself with 40 to 65 pounds for 8 miles. Chef and restaurateur Guy Fieri credits rucking as a key factor in his 30-pound weight loss. Country singer Brett Eldredge finds calm and clarity through weighted walks. You can do the same.

It might sound dramatic to say that rucking "saved" me, but shouldering the load helped me reclaim my sense of self, perseverance, and inner peace. Before rucking, I was stuck in a cycle of burnout and inconsistency, swinging between extremes—either all-in or all-out—letting all-or-nothing thinking get the best of me. Rucking helped me find the middle ground, keeping me engaged in the process. Like a good friend, rucking delivers what you need.

Whether it's challenge or comfort, you can tailor each ruck to yield your desired outcome; this book will teach you how.

Part One unpacks the physical and psychological benefits of rucking, while Part Two dives in to the how-to. You'll learn about essential gear, scalable training strategies, and how to care for your body from head to toe. Part Three details the importance of nutrition and mindset. You'll discover how to adapt your lifestyle to gain muscle and lose fat without feeling famished all the time. Insider tips from my work as a dietitian debunk decades of misleading nutrition guidelines and give you the confidence to get out and ruck and roll.

But first, let's lay some groundwork.

## WHAT IS RUCKING?

Rucking is walking or otherwise moving while carrying weight. Modern rucking involves loading a backpack with weight plates, sandbags, or anything heavy. It's walking, but way cooler—like "tactical" walking. If you've carried a backpack full of books or lugged around a baby, you've rucked.

The word *ruck* is both a noun and a verb. You can carry a ruck—short for "rucksack," which holds the weight—and you can go for a ruck. But don't confuse it with a ruck in rugby, when players from each team battle for possession of the ball. This book doesn't require a ball, and contact with other humans is optional.

Rucking is a straightforward way to challenge your cardiovascular system and stimulate muscle growth at the same time. It's not a replacement for weight training, but it makes an excellent beginner exercise if you enjoy walking and don't know how to start resistance training. Think of rucking as strength training for people who love cardio, and cardio for people who love strength training.

When wearing a ruck, the extra mass is on your torso, close to your center of gravity. This configuration transfers the load to larger muscle groups in your legs, back, and core so you build strength and endurance without extra strain on your feet and knees. Compared to running, rucking puts less force on joints while delivering similar benefits.[1] It works great for runners looking to build lower body strength because both running and rucking use many of the same muscles.

Carrying weight near your core is also safer compared to handheld or ankle weights (hello, 1980s!). Extra weight on the foot, such as with an ankle weight, is less efficient and places nine times more stress on joints versus carrying the same load on the torso. Weight carried in the hands—dumbbells, kettlebells, sandbags—disrupts arm swing and natural gait, forcing you to stray from natural locomotion. Smaller muscle groups in the hands and feet also fatigue faster, limiting the duration and intensity of a workout.[2] Rucking capitalizes on larger, stronger muscle groups, meaning you can exercise harder and longer with less risk of injury.

Because rucking activates muscles in the back and core, it can improve posture, which is especially beneficial for people with sedentary jobs or inactive lifestyles. Properly wearing a weighted pack corrects form by pulling back hunched shoulders and realigning the spine. Humans didn't evolve to sit all day. Our ancient ancestors walked long distances while carrying heavy loads. Rucking taps in to this primal movement, helping to correct the modern habit of sitting too much and moving too little, which wreaks havoc on our health.

Research shows that prolonged sitting increases the risk for chronic conditions such as obesity, type 2 diabetes, heart disease, and cancer. Sitting too much also deteriorates mental health, contributing to feelings of fatigue, anxiety, and depression. Americans today spend up to half (or more) of their waking hours seated, about 6½ to 8 hours, according to the Centers for Disease Control and Prevention (CDC).[3] Commuting, working a desk job, watching television, and even reading this book—the more you sit, the poorer your health outcomes.

According to the World Health Organization (WHO), physical inactivity ranks as the fourth leading risk factor for death, behind high blood pressure, tobacco use, and high blood sugar. A third of people worldwide don't meet the minimum recommendation of 150 minutes of moderate aerobic activity per week, which accounts for a whopping 3.2 million deaths annually. Dr. Rüdiger Krech, director of health promotion at the WHO, has called physical inactivity "a silent threat to global health."[4]

But the consequences go beyond mortality statistics. A sedentary lifestyle significantly degrades quality of life, raising the risk of developing musculoskeletal disorders such as poor bone density, low back pain, and knee pain. Ironically, these aches and pains become excuses to avoid exercise, even though incorporating more regular physical activity, not less, could largely prevent them. The good news? Even small bouts of exercise counteract these risks.

If you struggle with chronic arthritis or an autoimmune condition, don't dismiss the full-spectrum benefits of exercise, no matter how limited your ability. Any movement is better than none. Case in point: My husband, Jeremy, always physically capable and active, was diagnosed with fibromyalgia and rheumatoid arthritis, an autoimmune condition. The more he sits, the greater his pain. After months of crippling joint pain, insomnia, and no answers from specialists, he discovered that "motion is lotion." With low-impact activities, including rucking, he has adapted his movements to accommodate good days and bad. No two days play out the same, but everyone starts somewhere. Rucking could likewise help you get where you want to go.

The simplicity of rucking makes it an easy exercise for transitioning your body from static to strong. Start by just walking. After you've put some miles under your feet, add weight. Like walking, you can ruck anywhere, and you don't need fancy or expensive equipment to start. Ruck for free with items you already have on hand and upgrade your gear later. You just need a backpack, weight, and a sturdy pair of shoes.

One of rucking's greatest advantages is how easily you can adjust the intensity by varying the terrain, speed, and weight. Whether you're a beginner or experienced, you can personalize your workouts to suit your needs and goals. This book will help you get started (see Chapter 2 for progression strategies to help build stamina and strength, along with tips to help avoid injury). With a little trial and error, you'll discover what works best for you and enjoy the journey by going at your own pace.

Rucking offers something for everyone, from the solitude of solo adventure to the shared experience of group fitness. You can ruck alone, with friends, or as part of a local club that connects like-minded individuals. Like CrossFit, Peloton, and endurance running, the rucking community has a strong tribal culture, offering endless opportunities to test your limits, share progress, and celebrate milestones. It blends the independence of an individual pursuit with the camaraderie of a team sport.

Unlike many tech-driven fitness trends, rucking isn't about leaderboards, streaks, or gamifying your workout. There is no screen to distract you, and no competition is required. At its core, rucking has no rules, just a commitment to putting one foot in front of the other, regardless of how you carry the load.

# A BRIEF HISTORY OF RUCKING

Long before gyms and training protocols, humans carried heavy loads across expansive terrains. Homesteaders gathered water and food, hunters transported kills back to their communities, laborers carried tools and supplies to build civilizations, and soldiers bore gear into battle. Survival depended on walking and carrying, the essence of rucking.

During the Roman Empire, legionaries trained with loaded marches, walking nearly 20 miles while carrying around 20 kilograms, or about 45 pounds. For centuries, marching with packs has been a central part of military training, toughening troops for the physical and mental challenges of war. By the 1800s, standard military gear included knapsacks, later known as rucksacks, from the German *rücken,* meaning "back."

In more recent conflicts, combat loads ranged from 60 to 80 pounds. British soldiers in the Falklands War (1982) carried the heftiest rucks on record, averaging 50 kilograms (110 pounds). American troops in the Gulf Wars and Afghanistan also shouldered loads over 100 pounds. The ability to carry such heavy rucks doesn't happen overnight. Each military branch features boot camp training, where soldiers are sometimes required to carry up to half their body weight on a ruck march.[5]

One long-standing global endurance test is the Norwegian Foot March (NFM). Established in 1915, the NFM pushes both soldiers and civilians to their limits. Participants march for 30 kilometers (18.6 miles) while carrying a minimum of 11 kg (about 25 pounds), *excluding* water, food, or other consumables. Strictly monitored ruck weight must meet the minimum requirement at both the start and finish of the race. Military personnel must use military-approved rucksacks, while civilians can choose their preferred pack. Soldiers who complete the NFM within specific criteria—in uniform and between 4 hours 30 minutes and 6 hours, depending on age and gender—earn a Marsjmerket or "March" badge, one of the most difficult to attain. The Marsjmerket badge carries such prestige that American servicemen and women who achieve it may wear it on their military-issue uniform.[6]

Beyond the military, rucking has gained popularity among civilians. Ruck clubs and challenges such as the NFM highlight a growing social fitness movement, much like the rise of other foot races like 5Ks, 10Ks, and marathons. At the same time, rucking thrives as a solo pursuit, appealing to individuals interested in functional fitness, improving mental grit, and anyone looking to take their workout outdoors.

You can ruck for the health of it or ruck for the adventure of it. Ruck to prove your innate badassery, challenge yourself, or just to get out in nature. You don't need to carry an intimidating amount of weight to reap the benefits. In fact, I don't recommend it, especially when you're first starting out. Rucking is a scalable, approachable exercise that meets you where you're at and grows with you as you get stronger.

# MY JOURNEY

Before we jump in to the logistics, let me share the details of my journey—as a dietitian and a rucker—to offer camaraderie, hope, and inspiration, starting with my training as a dietitian.

In college, like many, I struggled with coursework, floundered between majors, and wrestled with how to fund it all. Pausing school to save money and inventory my options, I took a sales job. A few years later, I began studying to become a personal trainer, which was a personal passion, and I earned my certification within six months. Training others, however, made me neglect my own workouts, and the schedule of early mornings and late evenings proved exhausting. Dissatisfaction made me pivot toward nutrition. I realized I could help people improve their health through food, a path that instantly felt right for me.

Anyone who has searched for nutrition advice or Googled "how to lose weight" knows just how overwhelming and contradictory the information can be. Not to mention, we are notoriously unreliable at tracking what we eat. We underestimate portion sizes, misjudge how many calories we consume, and overestimate how much energy we burn. Food labels aren't much help either, with calorie counts that can vary by up to 20 percent, according to the FDA.[7] Countless other variables affect how we digest and use nutrients; it's no wonder why we feel lost. Sorting out the nutrition noise felt like meaningful work, and I knew I had found my calling.

I returned to college and persevered. In my last semester, I applied for highly competitive dietetic internships, and the prestigious Mayo Clinic in Rochester, Minnesota, my top choice, accepted my application. That yearlong experience became one of the most demanding and rewarding experiences of my life. It taught me that hospital work wasn't for me. Most patients didn't want to see a dietitian and complained about hospital food, rightfully so. But that program ignited my passion for outpatient education, where I could work with engaged people who were ready to learn.

After I passed my board exam and became a registered dietitian, reality hit hard. I prescribed low-fat diets for heart disease, low-sodium diets for high blood pressure, and carb-counting for people with diabetes, just like I was taught. I doled out 1,200-calorie meal plans like candy because that's what protocols told me to do. But my patients weren't thriving, and they deserved better. My directive to "eat less, move more" wasn't working for them, just as it hadn't worked for me in my own struggles with weight, emotional eating, and body image.

My professional training enabled me to roll up my sleeves and find out why. Every available strategy—Atkins, intermittent fasting, keto, paleo—gave me the opportunity to weigh the pros and cons of each approach. That's the beautiful frustration of nutrition: There's no one-size-fits-all answer. Like rucking, you have to find what works for you. Every lesson learned went into my toolbox, allowing me to help others build whole-life wellness plans customized to fit their needs. Real health doesn't force people into a rigid framework, it comes from building your own. It's a lesson I had to learn the hard way, and I use that experience today to help others create their own blueprint for real, sustainable results.

► ► ►

My discovery of rucking came later. In 2021, while I was driving to work, a massive wave of anxiety crashed over me. I gripped the steering wheel as an overwhelming sense of helplessness sank me into a panic. *I can't breathe, I can't drive.* My Apple Watch showed my heart rate soaring to 165 beats per minute, the equivalent of a hefty cardio session. But I was sitting in my car, motionless.

A battery of medical tests—ECG, chest X-rays, blood work—came back normal, but one finding stood out. The Generalized Anxiety Disorder-7 (GAD-7) screening tool assesses the severity of anxiety symptoms. Each question relates to a common symptom, such as feeling nervous, worrying too much, and having difficulty relaxing. Answers fall on a scale from 0 ("not at all") to 3 ("nearly every day"), resulting in a total score between 0 and 21. My score clocked in at 17, indicating severe anxiety. I had landed myself in the ER with my very first panic attack. After an uneventful run with a Holter monitor, my doctor immediately prescribed Prozac.

Prozac (fluoxetine) is a selective serotonin reuptake inhibitor (SSRI). SSRIs work by affecting a "feel-good" neurotransmitter linked to mood, sleep, pain, and appetite. Prozac and other SSRIs—including Zoloft (sertraline), Paxil (paroxetine), and Lexapro (escitalopram)—prevent nerve cells in the brain from reabsorbing serotonin too quickly. This action keeps serotonin in circulation, improving mood and (fingers crossed) reducing anxiety. But like any medication, SSRIs have side effects. Common side effects for SSRIs include nausea, drowsiness, insomnia, sexual dysfunction, and weight change. Prozac can't pick and choose which emotions to blunt, so some people (including me) experience an emotional flattening. Anxiety symptoms decline, but so do good emotions.

After six weeks on the medication, my GAD-7 score dropped from 17 to 7, from severe anxiety to mild. But this progress came at a cost. Similar to how the GAD-7 quantifies anxiety, the Patient Health Questionnaire-9 (PHQ-9) gauges the symptoms and severity of depression, and my PHQ-9 score was rising. Feelings of nervousness and worry yielded to new feelings of dissociation and apathy. The meds kicked me from one end of the spectrum to the other, from feeling everything to feeling nothing.

Once again, my medical training empowered me to find out why. Roughly 95 percent of serotonin is produced in your gut. In this gut-brain axis, food impacts mood and vice versa. But neither my own years of nutritional education nor my doctor addressed this important correlation. After my panic attack, my healthcare follow-ups didn't take exercise, sleep, or how I coped with stress into consideration. It turned out that my habit of drinking alcohol to "take the edge off" was *worsening* my anxiety.

The Alcohol and Drug Foundation describes hangover anxiety, or "hangxiety," as partly due to an imbalance of gamma-aminobutyric acid (GABA) and glutamate in the brain. Post-drinking anxiety is more likely to occur in people already suffering from anxiety, and hangxiety strikes in two ways. GABA, which promotes relaxation, increases with alcohol consumption. When you start drinking, a surge of GABA makes you feel calm. At the same time, alcohol suppresses glutamate, a chemical that makes your neurons fire, doubling booze's soothing effect. But this sedative effect lasts only so long.

After alcohol wears off, brain chemistry rebounds in the opposite direction. GABA plummets below baseline levels, replacing inhibition with agitation. Meanwhile, glutamate rises, leading to overstimulation of the nervous system. This double whammy creates a hyperactive brain state that often manifests as racing thoughts, heightened sensitivity, and increased anxiety.[8] As aphorist Mason Cooley said, "Alcohol postpones anxiety, then multiplies it."

The COVID-19 pandemic certainly didn't help matters. Many of us hunkered indoors, self-soothing with food and booze. We became increasingly sedentary as gyms locked up and the world locked down. Kitchens transformed into home offices, just an arm's length from the pantry and refrigerator. Nearly half of Americans reported weight gain, and folks with kids at home battled the bulge the most.[9] We jokingly named our collective weight gain the Quarantine 15. The inverse relationship between our waistlines and declining mental health became apparent, as fear and isolation became the "new norm." We ate and drank as a reward for surviving another day.

During the pandemic, women reported more frequent and heavier drinking.[10] Social distancing meant no social drinking, so we drank at home. I was no exception. At the end of the day, it wasn't a question of whether I was going to drink but *what* I was going to drink. My poor way of coping with the unrelenting strain of working in healthcare was wearing me down physically and emotionally. Something had to change.

In October 2021, I resigned from my role as a clinical dietitian, which unknowingly put me in the ranks of the great healthcare exodus. I was one of nearly 150,000 people who left their healthcare jobs in 2021 and 2022.[11] Stepping away from the clinic allowed me to go all-in with my own business. But this freedom came with its own challenges.

I didn't have a time clock to punch, so I burned the candle at both ends. Instead of banishing anxiety, these new circumstances shifted my worries. There was no longer a limit to how much I could work, and I didn't have the security of a regular salary. My self-worth became tied to my net worth. Toxic productivity made me feel lazy and undeserving whenever I wasn't *doing* something. A hustle-hard mentality—rise and grind; work hard, play hard; never stop—drove me into the ground. For entrepreneurs, burnout seemed like the norm. Quitting certainly wasn't an option, so the grind continued. My inner dialogue went uninterrupted with "shoulds." *I should be creating content. I should share this to social media. I should organize next month's calendar. I should log miles and prepare tax documents.*

When I did attempt to slow down, guilt and restlessness flooded my brain. Ignoring my own advice to engage in healthy behaviors, including sleeping, eating well, and exercising, made me feel like a hypocrite. Then I discovered rucking.

In 2022, on *The Drive* podcast, Peter Attia, MD, interviewed Michael Easter, who spoke openly about his struggle with alcohol. Easter's story shifted from sobriety to the benefits of boredom and spending time in nature. Attia and Easter discussed their hunting adventures and the pride that comes from doing hard things. Eventually, the conversation meandered into rucking and the benefits of walking with weight. This new-to-me form of fitness sounded great. Melt fat, build muscle, and increase bone density? Win, win, win.

So I started rucking, and the benefits of walking with weight took on another facet. Spending more time outdoors got me out of the house and out of my head. After a while, the physical benefits became secondary to the mental improvements. Rucking felt like nature's Prozac. It made me feel *good*: stronger, leaner, more clear-headed. The constant cloud of worry dissipated, which made me feel like me again. Each weighted step ironically made me feel lighter. Carrying something tangible on my shoulders helped me let go of what I'd been carrying psychologically. Rucking became my therapy, my relief, how I began reclaiming my mental health— one step at a time.

The activity soon became my new favorite exercise, which I recommended to others. Almost immediately, my inbox filled with questions: "How much weight should I start with?" "Can I ruck on a treadmill?" "What rucksack do you recommend?" (these questions and many others are addressed in Part Two).

Rucking quickly gained traction with my clients. A non-rucking foot injury sidelined Sarah, a client and busy mom of two young boys, who felt devastated when she had to pause the activity to heal. She described rucking as her "mental release" and scrambled for other ways to scratch the itch. Another client emailed a heartwarming note after her first ruck. After losing over 100 pounds, she picked up rucking, which caused her to reflect on her weight loss journey. Recognizing how challenging it felt to carry 10 extra pounds, she mentally teleported back to when her body carried more than 10 times that. It was a tangible reminder of her hard work and small daily choices that brought her to that moment, and she shed tears of joy at the realization.

Messages like that make my day. Rucking isn't a cure-all for life's hardships, but sharing the gospel of rucking allows me to pay it forward to others who might be struggling mentally or physically. While teaching a Rucking for Beginners class, I jokingly proclaimed it my life's mission to make sure that everyone tried rucking at least once. At the time, I never imagined this book as part of that declaration, so I'm grateful that you're here reading, learning, and, eventually, rucking.

Of course, imposter syndrome rears its ugly head for everyone at some point. In my case, that time is now. I've rucked for years not decades. I don't have a magazine-worthy physique, and I'm not particularly athletic. I'm average in many ways. I ruck for the health of it, but that's exactly the point. I want you to have a down-to-earth, practical resource that can benefit you, regardless of your fitness level. I hope rucking gives you a new, healthier way to manage stress, get out of your head, and get into nature.

If, like me, you love to walk but feel like it's not enough, you'll love rucking. No more guilt for "just" walking when you can make the most of each step by adding a little extra weight. You can tailor your rucks to be as easy or hard as you like. You don't have to drive to a gym or buy fancy equipment. That's one of my favorite features of rucking. It's highly customizable and accessible to nearly everyone.

But don't let the simplicity fool you. Rucking capitalizes on the simplest, most fundamental forms of movement—walking and carrying—which help you achieve tough goals too. GORUCK, a company founded by former Green Beret Jason McCarthy, is built around this very idea. Known for its durable gear and global ruck club network and events, GORUCK recognizes the physical and mental advantages of the sport. As McCarthy says, "Do hard things, and the rest of life gets easier."

Rucking is more than a workout; it's a metaphor for life itself. Some days, the load feels heavy, like the weight of the world on your shoulders; other days, it feels light and easy. Whether you're physically underworked or mentally overwhelmed—or gripping the steering wheel of life, like I was—learning to carry the load will help you appreciate the strength in the struggle and achieve your full potential.

Thank you for joining the *Ruck Fit* community by reading this book and learning how to make the most of each step. Let's get to it!

## REMEMBER

► Rucking is walking or moving with weight. All you need is a backpack, something heavy, and sturdy shoes. (See Chapter 3 for more on gear.)

► Rucking combines endurance and strength training, but it's not a replacement for weight lifting.

► Rucking originates from military training, but the essence of rucking dates back thousands of years as a cornerstone of human evolution and survival.

# PART ONE

# The Benefits of Rucking

# 1

Small Steps,
Big Gains

If you don't make time for exercise,
you'll probably have to make time for illness.

—ROBIN SHARMA,
AUTHOR AND LEADERSHIP EXPERT

n today's fast-paced, developed societies, the demands of daily life overshadow the link between physical and mental well-being. Inactivity has become so routine that most people overlook its transformative effects on their own health and happiness. We spend nearly 90 percent of our day indoors, trading sunlight and fresh air for screens and climate-controlled spaces.[12]

We look in awe at folks who run in cold weather or make it to the gym on Fridays or holidays. We should emulate that behavior, though, because the research is clear: Our bodies, designed for movement, thrive in the natural world. Neglecting these needs affects more than just our physical fitness. Lack of movement and not spending time in nature damages mental clarity, emotional resilience, and overall quality of life. When we move better, we live better, unlocking physical vitality, mental sharpness, and a renewed connection to ourselves and the world around us.

This chapter explains why you should give a ruck about rucking and how prioritizing your physical and mental fitness transforms your life. You don't need to become an endurance athlete or ruck hard every day to reap the benefits. This isn't about extremes. It's about embracing small, consistent steps that add up to meaningful change. Movement, even in its simplest form, can set the stage for a healthier, more resilient you. It's time to break the cycle and take control—not tomorrow, not next month. *Today*.

# THE COST OF COMFORT

Humans are wired to choose easy. To conserve energy, our brains automatically resist change. Seeking comfort isn't a form of laziness—it's biology. This survival mechanism kept our ancestors alive during times of scarcity, when conserving energy meant they were more likely to find food, avoid danger, and care for their communities long enough to pass on their genes. But in today's world of endless convenience, that same biology can work against us, keeping us glued to the couch when what we really need is to move.

For example, feeding ourselves—once a labor-intensive, community-driven undertaking—has become as simple as walking or driving to a grocery store and putting prepackaged foods in a wheeled shopping cart and onto a conveyor belt. We have the added luxury of getting food delivered right to our front door. We have taxis or ride-sharing services if we don't want to walk. We work remote jobs so we don't have to leave the house. We accomplish most everything we need to without ever stepping outside or interacting with another human being.

Technology allows us to check chat messages, emails, texts, or all three at once. Smartphones—intentionally engineered with the same addictive mechanics as slot machines—buzz with a dopamine drip of notifications that distract us from developing or maintaining deep, personal connections with other people. The average American spends half the day staring at a screen, sometimes "double-screening," viewing two screens simultaneously, such as streaming TV while scrolling social media on a phone or tablet. Baby boomers average around three hours of screen time, while Gen Z exceeds seven hours per day.[13] The rise in screen time doesn't just drain batteries—it zaps your energy too.

Healthy living takes effort. Exercising, cooking nutritious meals, and not doomscrolling all benefit us in the long term, but we often find them hard to maintain in the short term. It's simpler and more satisfying to tap a device, swipe a screen, and click a button for instant gratification. But if you want to thrive, not just survive, you must push beyond immediate discomfort. Unfortunately, we take this idea to the extreme by setting big fitness goals—like working out an hour per day, every day—can feel overwhelming and unsustainable. Unrealistic expectations about exercising enough to make it "count" keep us from taking meaningful action. When the goal feels too daunting, we give up before we even start.

The price for our collective lack of physical activity is staggering: an estimated $117 billion in annual healthcare costs. More than 10 percent of premature deaths correlate to a lack of movement.[14] Exercise outperforms numerous medications for blood pressure, diabetes, and other conditions, but so many of us opt out of this free, effective tool. Despite the well-documented benefits, we choose convenience and comfort.

Then a life-altering health diagnosis strikes. Despite not eating well or exercising, we wonder, *Why me?* As author Bill Bryson grimly observed in *The Body*, "Suicide by lifestyle takes ages." Muscle and bone atrophy when you don't use them, and a sedentary life lead to less strength, more fragility, and declining health.

Blood sugar rises, and inflammation spikes, beckoning the 35 chronic diseases associated with inactivity.[15] We bargain with ourselves, kicking the can down the road. *I'll start tomorrow, Monday, or next month.* Convenience triumphs over health once again, pulling another brick from the wall of what could be good health.

Here's the thing: Any movement is better than none. A few stretches, a short walk, or a light ruck can shift your mindset and your health. Small steps can lead to big changes over time. It's true, there's no such thing as a bad workout. Sure, you might not do all that you wanted or planned, but doing something is better than doing nothing. Movement and exercise change the game. Prioritizing physical fitness, including activities such as rucking, ultimately leads to a longer, healthier life.

When movement forms part of your daily life, you metabolize food better, sleep more soundly, and experience less inflammation. How? Muscle. It's not just about brute strength or looking "toned." Muscle matters for your health, vitality, and longevity. Let's take a closer look.

## THE POWER OF MUSCLE

Strong, active muscles lift heavy objects, but they also function as the body's metabolic powerhouses. They help stabilize blood sugar, reduce the risk of metabolic disorders, and produce hormones that counteract inflammation and boost mood. On the flip side, weak or underused muscles can lead to a cascade of problems: fatigue, stress, joint pain, and increased vulnerability to chronic health conditions. Diminished strength and a sedentary lifestyle create a vicious spiral, seeping into our mental health and fueling frustration, anxiety, and depression. Breaking free from this cycle begins with just one step.

By prioritizing regular movement and building strength,

you can unlock a path to physical resilience, mental clarity, and a renewed sense of control over your health. Muscle mass and function predict quantity and quality of life, meaning how long (lifespan) and how well (health span) you live. Physical fitness improves resiliency and minimizes frailty that can accompany aging or follow illness and injury.[16] Many of us aim to live longer and accept declining health as an inevitable part of aging. We envision retirement as a time to travel or enjoy life's luxuries, yet many of us will have surpassed peak physical fitness by then. But loss of strength and vitality isn't an unavoidable fate—it's a choice.

Muscle is about so much more than looking good. It allows you to live independently: to bathe, dress, and feed yourself; to get in and out of bed or a chair unassisted; to manage your personal hygiene and other activities of daily living (ADLs). These "little" things *are* the big things. Consider that 10 percent of people over age 75 require help with basic ADLs. By age 85, that number doubles.[17]

Aging is a natural process, yes, but loss of function is optional. Regular exercise can help mitigate physical and cognitive decline. If you've cared for or witnessed a loved one endure this decline, you know how heartbreaking it is for everyone involved. To avoid this fate for yourself, you need to build a reserve of physical strength and mental resilience. Rucking can help you achieve both.

## METABOLIC HEALTH

How well your cellular machinery operates constitutes metabolic health. The quality of your metabolic health determines how efficiently your body is able to break down and process food and toxins, transport nutrients and signals to the proper places, and build and repair tissues. It's more than how many calories you burn and includes how well your body adapts to stress. Because metabolic health involves so many different systems, the term doesn't have an official definition, but we do have criteria to diagnose *metabolic syndrome*.

Metabolic syndrome is a cluster of symptoms often stemming from insulin resistance, which leads to impaired metabolic function, including poor blood sugar control. As with the early stages of diabetes, many folks don't even know they have metabolic syndrome. So how do you know if you do? The following checklist summarizes research from three of the world's leading health organizations: the World Health Organization (WHO), International Diabetes Federation (IDF), and National Cholesterol Education Program (NCEP). Three or more of the following symptoms indicate the presence of metabolic syndrome, most of which are evaluated during an annual physical. Which of these apply to you?

**Elevated fasting glucose:** 100+ mg/dL, on medication for high blood sugar, or diagnosed with diabetes

**High triglycerides:** 150+ mg/dL or on medication to treat elevated triglycerides

**Low HDL cholesterol:** <35–40 mg/dL in men and <40–50 mg/dL in women or on medication to treat low HDL

**High blood pressure:** >130/85 mmHg or on medication to treat hypertension

**Large waist circumference:** Waist-to-hip ratio 0.9+ for men or 0.85+ for women or BMI over 30 kg/m2 (WHO); waist circumference 94–102+ cm (37–40 in.) for men and 80–88+ cm (32–35 in.) for women (IDF, NCEP)

Carrying excess weight around the middle raises the risk of metabolic syndrome and often signals the presence of visceral fat—a harmful type of fat that surrounds and infiltrates vital organs. Even just a little fat around the liver, for instance, can wreak metabolic misery on the body, exacerbating insulin resistance. In sedentary individuals, fat can also work its way into muscle tissue, disrupting its function. While metabolic syndrome and obesity mirror each other, they're not the same. Many diagnostically "obese" people are metabolically healthy, and many people with "normal" BMIs have metabolic syndrome. Like rucking, it's not about the weight but how you carry it.

Physical activity can help prevent metabolic syndrome. Building and preserving muscle with exercise positively impacts metabolic health by reversing insulin resistance, restoring mitochondrial function, reducing inflammation, enhancing metabolic flexibility, and increasing bone health. The remainder of this chapter delves in to the specific health benefits of rucking. Before we dive in, it's important to acknowledge how little research we have on rucking for the general population, particularly women. Rucking originated in the military, so most research studies have followed young, fit men carrying obscene amounts of weight. We need more data, but in the meantime, we can compile the real-world experiences of everyday people, just like you, whom I've interviewed in the course of my work.

# IMPROVE CARDIOVASCULAR FITNESS

A low-impact, steady state (LISS) exercise, rucking provides a manageable level of intensity that can suit your current fitness level while still challenging your heart and lungs. As you build aerobic fitness, you can modify your rucks to support improvements in your cardiovascular health to reap greater fitness gains (more about that in Chapter 2).

Regular rucking improves heart health, boosts endurance, builds stamina, and conditions the body to handle prolonged exercise, making it easier to conquer everyday activities. Improving cardiovascular fitness makes your body more efficient at transporting oxygen, resulting in better blood pressure control and enhanced lung function. Climbing stairs or carrying groceries will feel easier, and you'll feel stronger during workouts.

Training zones provide a simple way to categorize difficulty of exertion. Depending on the source, zones range according to heart rate, effort, and, in more technical cases, blood lactate. They scale from very light activity (Zone 1) to maximum effort (Zone 5). Here's a simple breakdown of each level, based on what's known as the talk test.

**Zone 1:** Easy, low-intensity activity that promotes circulation without strain. Zone 1 includes warm-ups, cooldowns, and rest-day activities. At this effort, you can speak comfortably in complete sentences.

**Zone 2:** Low-to-moderate intensity, with mild strain that feels sustainable for more than an hour. You can maintain a conversation, but someone would know that you're exercising.

**Zone 3:** Moderate-to-high effort. Breathing becomes labored, transferring from your nose to mouth, and it's harder to talk.

**Zone 4:** High-intensity effort often used for interval training to build speed and power. Breathing becomes difficult, and you can speak only a few words at a time.

**Zone 5:** All-out efforts at peak performance. Your respiratory system is working at max capacity, and you feel breathless. Conversation isn't possible.

Zone 2, where most people ruck under light load, on flat terrain, provides the ideal balance of challenge and sustainability. It's the sweet spot for building a cardiovascular base. It requires gentle effort but still offers significant gains in aerobic fitness and metabolic health. As your conditioning progresses, you'll be able to tolerate higher intensities while maintaining a conversational Zone 2 pace. In other words, the huffing and puffing you experience during your first ruck will eventually feel like a breeze as your heart and lungs become more efficient. No zone is better than another, though. It's normal to fluctuate between zones and intensities, especially when rucking outside on unpredictable terrain. All zones provide cardiovascular benefits, and any exercise is better than none, especially when you're first starting out.

# BUILD MUSCLE AND CORE STRENGTH

Rucking strengthens the back, shoulders, legs, and abdomen. It counteracts the effects of sitting too much, building a stronger core that supports the spine and reduces the risk of lower back pain. Consider rucking the antidote to sitting.

Like any exercise, maintaining good form will help avoid injury and maximize benefits. Start with manageable weight and focus on your posture to build strength and reinforce your natural movement patterns. Carrying too much weight too fast will cause discomfort or injury.

While rucking helps increase muscle mass, it won't make you look bulky, and it isn't a substitute for weight training. Women, who naturally have lower bone density and muscle mass compared to men, have the most to gain from rucking. In fact, women have a leg up when it comes to the exercise. Typically, women have a lower center of gravity, giving them more stability under load.

They also have a higher proportion of slow-twitch muscle fibers, which resist fatigue, allowing them to sustain longer efforts with greater endurance.

In Michael Easter's book *The Comfort Crisis*, Jason McCarthy explains how rucking builds a "supermedium" body type: not too skinny, not too muscular. He notes that, in the military, being too big slows people down, so rucking is a great way to correct for body type. If you're carrying extra fluff, rucking can lean you out. If you're skinnier than you'd like, rucking can help you gain muscle mass—but that's not all.

# BURN MORE CALORIES

Building muscle not only results in a greater calorie burn at rest, it also gives you the strength and power to push harder during workouts, meaning you'll burn more calories during exercise, too. Depending on load, elevation, speed, and other variables, rucking can burn up to two or three times more calories than walking.[18] [19]

To compare the difference between a 1-mile walk and a 1-mile ruck, I tracked both workouts using my Apple Watch. I followed the same flat, paved route and kept the same workout time, distance, and pace. Only the load changed. Here are the results:

|  | Workout time | Distance | Pace | Average HR | Calorie burn |
|---|---|---|---|---|---|
| Walk | 21:14 | 1.12 miles | 18:58 | 118 | 118 |
| Ruck with 20 pounds | 21:15 | 1.12 miles | 18:58 | 143 | 176 |

My average heart rate increased by about 20 percent, and my calorie burn jumped by half. Fitness trackers can prove inaccurate, but it's still fun to compare the data for yourself. If you don't have a wearable fitness tracker, use an online calculator to estimate your calorie burn during a ruck. GORUCK, for example, has a rucking calorie calculator (goruck.com/pages/rucking-calorie-calculator). Enter your body weight, ruck weight, pace, and grade to estimate your burn.

*Outside* (OutsideOnline.com) also offers a digital backpacking calorie estimator using the Pandolf equation. Enter your body weight, pack weight, speed, slope, and terrain (paved road, gravel road, sand, and the like) to generate your calorie burn per hour or mile. The Pandolf equation underestimates calories burned under load,[20] but calorie calculators are for estimation purposes only. Actual results depend on body composition, physical fitness, and changes in elevation or terrain.

Calories aside, physical activity increases your capacity for glucose uptake and improves insulin sensitivity. That means carbs won't spike your blood sugar into the stratosphere (especially if you ruck after a meal), and you become more metabolically flexible. Metabolic flexibility refers to how efficiently you can switch between burning glucose and fat. People with high metabolic flexibility adapt more easily to different diets, exercise intensities, and fasting states without major disruptions.

On the flip side—when inflammation riddles your body, excess fat encases your liver, or you have low muscle tone—the switch from burning glucose to fat becomes more difficult. You struggle to make it more than a few hours without eating. You might also experience intense cravings (especially for carbs or sugar), energy crashes, irritability, and mood swings.

Think of muscle as a sponge for circulating blood sugar. The more muscle you have, the more glucose you can absorb. Maintaining stable blood sugar in healthy ranges douses inflammation, making it easier for your body's systems to do their work efficiently and avoid the unpleasant symptoms of poor metabolic flexibility.

# SLOW BONE LOSS AND PREVENT FRAILTY

Walking with weight can improve bone density, reducing the risk of fractures and frailty. Bone breaks can lead to muscular imbalances and decreased independence for daily activities. For an elderly person, a broken bone, especially a hip, can prove life-threatening. Many people recover from bone fractures without any problems, but for older folks, a broken bone can be the beginning of the end. Moving less contributes to muscle loss, which degrades metabolic health. Limited mobility also increases social isolation, affecting mental health, too. Up to 20 percent of aging people who break a hip die within one year, and another 50 percent require extra help to function.[21]

Osteopenia is the medical term for moderate total bone loss. Osteoporosis describes a more advanced stage of bone loss, in which bones become brittle, porous, and prone to fractures. A bone mineral density (BMD) test helps diagnose both conditions, often with a dual-energy X-ray absorptiometry (DEXA) scan. The resulting T-score compares your BMD to that of a young healthy adult, while a Z-score shows how you compare to others of the same age and gender.

**Normal:** T-score above -1

**Osteopenia:** T-score between -1.0 and -2.5

**Osteoporosis:** T-score of -2.5 or lower

Peak bone mass occurs between ages 30 and 35, but if you're older than that, it's not too late to intervene. Bone isn't static tissue; it's constantly building up and breaking down. Rucking creates mechanical stress on the body, which initiates bone growth. According to Wolff's Law, a principle of bone theory, bones adapt to the mechanical force they encounter. Regular weight-bearing exercise, such as from rucking (but not swimming, for example), strengthens bones to better handle the load.

Exercise alone can't maximize bone health, though. You must provide a consistent supply of essential building blocks: protein, calcium, magnesium, vitamin D, and other vital nutrients. If you ruck outdoors, sun exposure helps facilitate vitamin D production. Vitamin D increases calcium absorption in the digestive tract which, in turn, aids bone development.

Bone health matters, especially for women after menopause. As estrogen levels plummet, bone breakdown outpaces bone building. The good news is progressive resistance training can increase BMD in postmenopausal women by 1 to 4 percent each year.[21] More on how to do that with rucking in the next chapter.

Julie, 61, from southwest Florida, received a diagnosis of osteoporosis, and she panicked after her doctor warned her not to fall. She couldn't run, do HIIT workouts, or CrossFit—all good for improving bone density but too risky. She didn't want to take medication or join a gym, so she did her research and discovered rucking. She already had a daily walking routine, so she added weight along with low-impact strength exercises and yoga. Her next DEXA scan showed improvement in her T-scores. Now she feels like "a million bucks," and her doctor said, "Keep doing what you're doing!"

# REDUCE ANXIETY AND DEPRESSION

Rucking relieves stress and stimulates the release of endorphins. These neurotransmitters create a sense of well-being, similar to a "runner's high" but with less impact on your joints.

For example, Sarah experiences a "rucker's high." Now 18 years sober, she turned to running during her early days of sobriety. When she couldn't run, she tried rucking and was thrilled to find a low-impact activity that provided the same psychological perks. She also reports generating her best ideas while rucking, which she attributes to phone-free exercise. Tech timeouts like this offer another unquestionably effective strategy to improve mental health.

Many people turn to rucking not just for fitness, but for the mental clarity it brings. Sam from Texas beautifully articulates the correlation between rucking and depression: "Depression feels heavy and makes it feel like every step, every motion, takes more effort—kind of like rucking. At least with a ruck on, I can focus on taking the next step. Step forward, repeat. Every time I finish a ruck, I get to say 'Suck it, Depression. I'm moving forward.'" Each time you complete a ruck, you can claim the same victory.

Doing hard things, whether it's fighting the gravitational pull of your couch or completing a tough ruck, creates a sense of accomplishment. With each step, your confidence grows, reinforcing positive self-image and reducing feelings of anxiety and self-doubt. You reclaim the mental bandwidth to overcome life's inevitable challenges, becoming better suited to prevail when adversity strikes. Better yet, you don't have to go at it alone.

## CULTIVATE SOCIAL CONNECTIONS

Whether in a local club, fitness group, or spontaneous gathering of friends, rucking with others can improve your psychological well-being. A sense of belonging matters critically for individuals and society at large, especially as we grapple with the epidemics of loneliness and physical inactivity. Rucking with others creates accountability, motivating you to show up for yourself and the group. Shared camaraderie generates excitement and encouragement to face new challenges. At the same time, everyone in the group enjoys a customized experience. Whether you're a beginner or an experienced athlete, rucking lets everyone carry a weight that works for them while still moving together. Everyone gets a good workout, and no one feels left behind. Everyone wins.

Research also suggests that walking in the same direction with someone—a friend, spouse, colleague—builds a sense of unity and can disarm charged conversations.[22] Build bonds and solve problems by walking together . . . with weight.

To connect with like-minded individuals, search the GORUCK directory (goruck.com) for a list of more than 500 ruck clubs that are easily searchable by state. If you can't find a local group, start your own—like I did. All you need is a gathering place to tell people where you'll be rucking and when. Create a social media page or start a group text with family or friends. Then go outside and get after it.

# RECONNECT WITH NATURE

In a world dominated by screens and indoor living, reconnecting with nature is more than a luxury—it's a necessity. Getting outside contributes to positive mental health in many ways. Rucking qualifies as a "green exercise"—physical activity performed in natural environments such as parks, forests, or trails. Independently, exercise and spending time in nature reduce stress, improve attention span, and boost self-esteem. Combine them for even greater benefit.[23]

Even if you don't live near scenic trails, you can benefit from rucking outside. Daylight exposure can realign your body's circadian rhythm, the internal clock that regulates sleep, energy levels, and metabolism. Before the lightbulb, the sun started and ended our day, dictating how we lived. Today, the average person spends more than 90 percent of the day indoors, under artificial light. Regular sunlight exposure normalizes your circadian rhythm, so you release melatonin at the optimal time, reinforcing quality sleep. Sunlight also boosts serotonin, the "feel-good" neurotransmitter that many antidepressants and antianxiety medications target. Rucking outside will help reset your internal clock naturally, supporting better sleep and overall well-being.

# EMBRACE MINDFULNESS

Every ruck gives you an opportunity to clean house mentally. Tech-free rucking means focusing on your posture, breath, steps, and surroundings. If you're concerned about safety, you can of course take your device with you. But turn your phone off or put it in airplane mode and stow it in your pack—out of sight.

Spending time in nature always leaves me with a sense of awe and wonder. Minnesota experiences all the seasons, and phone-free rucking allows me to appreciate each of them. Witnessing nature's cycles helps remind me of life's interconnectedness. Pause and savor the peace and clarity of your own surroundings. Even in the suburbs or a big city, you can observe the scenery around you. Rucking can turn familiar streets or parks into spaces of discovery. You might spot subtle details that escaped you before, like a neighbor's quirky garden gnome or a local business you hadn't noticed.

In this sense, rucking is a holistic way to strengthen your body, calm your mind, and reconnect with yourself and the environment around you. The cumulative benefits build a stronger, more resilient version of you—inside and out.

## REMEMBER

- Modern-day conveniences make it easy to fall victim to comfort. If you want to thrive, not just survive, you must exercise regularly.
- Muscle makes the magic happen. It stabilizes blood sugar levels, improves metabolic health, and counteracts inflammation.
- Walking with weight can improve bone density and reduce the risk of frailty and fractures, helping to preserve independence.
- Rucking in nature has physical and mental benefits. It burns more calories than walking, builds muscle and endurance, and reduces anxiety, depression, and loneliness.

# PART TWO

# How to Ruck

# 2

## Getting Started

In truth, one step at a time is not too difficult.

—OG MANDINO, AUTHOR OF
*THE GREATEST SALESMAN IN THE WORLD*

This chapter covers everything you need to start rucking today, including tips for beginners, answers to common questions, and other practical advice. You'll learn how to find the sweet spot of staying challenged without overdoing it. You'll explore progression techniques and strategies to prevent injuries, including how to distinguish between discomfort and pain, so you can test your limits safely and effectively.

But first, an important note. As with any new exercise, consider your current fitness level and limitations. Whether you're new to fitness or looking for a fresh challenge, rucking offers a low-barrier entry to functional training, but it requires checking your ego at the door. You might feel tempted to max out your load or tackle long distances right off the bat, but too much too soon increases the risk of injuries, including blisters, muscle strains, and even stress fractures. Start light, take it slow, and listen to your body as you build strength and stamina over time.

# WALK FIRST, THEN RUCK

If you lead a mostly sedentary life, walk before you ruck. Before you add weight, you must establish a consistent walking habit first. Walking improves joint mobility, reinforces gait and balance, and prepares you to walk under load. Without that foundation, you could sustain injury from improper form, overuse, or any other setback. There's no sense in taking one step forward and two steps back.

In America, the average adult walks less than 5,000 steps per day (compare that to our hunter-gatherer ancestors who walked an estimated 10,000 to 18,000 steps per day). If you're a beginner, aim for 5,000 to 7,000 steps per day, a reasonable baseline goal. Gradually work up to a number that challenges you but doesn't feel daunting. Studies suggest that anywhere from 4,000 to 12,000 steps per day significantly lowers the risk of premature death and improves overall health.[24] For example, as little as 3,500 steps per day have been shown to prevent people with prediabetes from making the jump to full-blown type 2 diabetes.[25] If you're pursuing weight management and increased cardiovascular fitness, aim for a bit more, 10,000 to 12,000 steps daily. But don't expect to hit those numbers overnight.

Begin by observing your current daily step count. Use a smartphone or fitness tracker to find your average daily steps across a week. You can also use a pedometer app or an old-fashioned, clip-on pedometer to monitor your steps.

Once you have your average step count, increase it by 10 to 20 percent each week until you consistently reach 7,500 to 12,000 steps per day with good form. Step goals will vary from person to person, so adjust the goal based on your starting point.

If you want to jump in to rucking, walk with an empty backpack or a light load—no more than 10 or 15 pounds—as you increase your steps gradually. Step count naturally fluctuates from day to day, so focusing on a weekly average will help you stay on track without getting preoccupied with daily numbers. For example, if you hit 12,000 steps one day and 8,000 another, that's right on target for a daily goal of 10,000 steps. Don't overthink it—every step counts.

Seasonal weather can make it hard to muster the will to walk or ruck. In freezing winter wind, relentless spring rain, or sweltering summer heat, it's more comfortable to stay indoors. But training in diverse conditions builds toughness and unlocks biological benefits. Cold exposure stimulates metabolism and improves resilience, whereas heat acclimation enhances cardiovascular efficiency. So dress appropriately and embrace the suck. The benefits of rucking in the elements might surprise you. For example, rucking in the rain means no bugs swarming your face. On winter rucks, you'll warm up much faster when you're wearing weight and, again, no bugs! (Chapter 3 explores specific gear and strategies for rucking in hot and cold weather.)

If you have a hard time reaching your goals, try these year-round tips to boost your step count:

- After every meal, take a walk, even if it's just a short one.
- Take the stairs instead of the elevator.
- Install a walking pad (the bottom part of a treadmill) under your standing desk.
- Walk or ruck while on phone calls or during meetings.
- Whether at home or in the office, use the farthest bathroom, printer, or water fountain from your workstation.
- Every hour or every time you get up to use the restroom, walk 5 to 10 times around your office, living room, or kitchen.
- Vacuum and tackle other step-heavy chores around your home.
- Walk on a treadmill or walking pad while watching TV.
- Shop in stores or malls instead of online.
- If you drive anywhere, park as far from the entrance to your destination as possible.

Being intentional about how and when you move, even on busy days, benefits your health. Every step counts, so start small and stay consistent.

# CARRY THE LOAD

Once you have some miles under your feet and have built a solid walking habit, begin with a light load. Most people can begin rucking comfortably with 10 to 20 pounds, typically 10 to 15 pounds for women and 15 to 20 pounds for men. Your fitness level, physical limitations, and environment will influence your starting weight. Adjust the weight up or down, as needed, to bear the load without risking injury. You can add more weight later, but you can't undo an injury. If in doubt, err on the side of caution and start light. And always be aware of any mobility challenges you may have and consult your doctor if you're not sure whether an activity is right for you.

You can use almost anything heavy to start. Load a backpack with textbooks, water bottles, bricks, or even rocks—literally "rocking." When I started rucking, I wrapped a 10-pound dumbbell in a bath towel and stuffed it in an old backpack. After enjoying the activity consistently enough to invest in quality gear, I purchased cast-iron weight plates that felt more comfortable and allowed me to carry heavier loads. As the weight increases, you will likely need sturdier equipment. More on gear in Chapter 3.

After the first ruck or two, most people increase weight pretty quickly. In my case, 10 pounds felt easy enough to carry, though a new tightness developed in my hips, which came from the change in posture. While the weight may feel light, learning how your body adapts under load matters just as much. Your ability to maintain good posture indicates that you're using the right amount of weight. You should be able to walk upright, without hunching forward. Leaning forward means you're carrying too much. The weight should feel secure and not bounce around in your pack or against your back. Center the load securely on your upper back to avoid strain or injury. Don't let it sag toward your butt or rest on your lower back. Like a military haircut, you want to secure the load "high and tight" for optimal comfort and safety.

As you build strength and endurance, add weight in increments of 5 to 10 pounds. Early in your rucking journey, an extra 5 pounds can feel like 20, so always plan a short ruck to test the new load. You can also add smaller amounts of weight. Formal weights usually come in 5-pound increments, so if you want to go lighter than that, you may have to get creative by using odds and ends, such as a can of beans (1 pound), a large hardcover book (2 pounds), or a bag of rice (variable).

Eventually, you'll find your base weight, a midrange amount that feels comfortably uncomfortable. For heavy rucks, add 5 to 15 pounds, making sure, again, to shorten the distance or duration to avoid injury. Remove weight for a light ruck, like when you're navigating new terrain with lots of elevation or you feel depleted from consecutive training days.

The gold standard is to work up to carrying 25 to 30 percent of your body weight, with a limit of 50 pounds. Progression takes time—months or even years—so practice patience. Rucking itself isn't a race. Sarah's advice to new ruckers: "There's no rush. Add weight, and if it feels funky, unadd it or go for a short ruck."

Not everyone will max out by carrying 30 percent of their body weight, though. Many women, including me, feel comfortable with a base weight of 20 to 25 pounds. Even if you don't reach that threshold, you still reap the benefits. On the other hand, if you hit 30 percent of your body weight and feel it's manageable, you can challenge your fitness in other ways, with some methods being more effective than weight alone. More on those strategies later in the chapter.

## TIPS FOR BEGINNERS

Rucking races exist, but the activity itself isn't a competition. It's about building strength and resilience at your own pace. As your body adapts, rucks feel easier as you get stronger. To help scale your workouts and find what works best for you, let's review a few key concepts to help you get started.

**Begin with a short ruck.** Walk no more than 1 or 2 miles at first, to see how your body responds. When you're starting out, try rucking just twice per week, with two recovery days between sessions.

**Change one variable at a time.** For safe, sustainable progress, increase weight, distance, duration, speed, or incline gradually and individually—never more than one element at once. If a ruck feels too easy, change *only one* variable the next time. If you ruck too heavy, too long, too often, or all of the above, you'll diminish your gains. Limit yourself to no more than one strenuous ruck—or "sucky ruck," as I like to call them—per week. These longer, heavier outings push your limits and can "hurt so good." A little of that goes a long way.

**Mix it up.** If you plan to make rucking your primary source of cardio, diversify your week: one light ruck, two or three moderate rucks with your base weight, and one sucky ruck. Pair with resistance training, mobility work, and rest days to compound your gains without causing injury. See Chapter 4 for sample workout schedules.

▶ ▶ ▶

Before we dive in to common questions, let's recap some beginner tips to help you avoid newbie pitfalls.

**Take it easy.** Start light. Go slow. Walk short distances. Stay on flat ground.

**Secure the load.** Keep the weight high and tight on your back.

**Focus on form.** Be mindful of posture and engage your core to walk fully upright. If you're leaning forward, you're carrying too much weight.

**Don't ruck too much.** Avoid rucking more than three days per week at first.

**Keep it simple.** Don't get stuck by analysis paralysis. Load your pack, head outside, and learn as you go.

Now that you have a solid foundation, let's tackle some frequently asked questions to fine-tune your approach and maximize your results.

# ANSWERS TO COMMON QUESTIONS

Despite the simplicity of walking with weight, rucking comes with lots of questions, especially from beginners. Let's answer some common questions to help make your journey as seamless as possible.

▶ *What's the difference between rucking and hiking?*
While both activities involve walking outdoors and offer cardiovascular benefits, they differ in purpose and intensity. Hiking typically focuses on recreation and enjoying a leisurely journey through nature. Rucking emphasizes a consistent, moderate pace and involves more than carrying snacks and day-hike essentials. You go out of your way to bear extra load when you ruck, rather than

look for ways to cut weight as backpackers often do. The challenge of rucking comes from the added weight, whereas with hiking, the difficulty usually lies in the terrain. You can easily transform a hike into a ruck by packing more than water, food, and bug spray. Pack an extra weight plate *on purpose*, and now you're rucking. Hiking tends to take place in scenic landscapes, such as woods, trails, or mountains. But you can ruck pretty much anywhere: around the block, down the street, in a mall, even at the gym.

▶ *How can I track a ruck on my smart watch or fitness tracker?*
Most fitness trackers don't have an option to track rucking (yet), but you can hack this in one of two ways. If you're walking on relatively flat ground, track the ruck as you would a regular walk. For steeper terrain with more hills, track the ruck as a hike to reflect the greater demand. If your device has a built-in heart rate monitor, it should recognize the increased intensity. RuckWell and other free apps also track stats and estimate calorie burn.

Fitness trackers provide useful approximations, but they aren't 100 percent accurate, especially with calories. Use the data as a ballpark estimation rather than a precise measurement.

▶ *Can I ruck too much? Can I ruck every day?*
Yes, you can ruck too much. Theoretically, you *could* ruck every day—as long as you're not rucking heavy every day. Remember the law of diminishing returns: More isn't always better. Rucking, though a versatile exercise, won't meet all your fitness needs. It can't replace strength training, and your overall fitness routine should incorporate a healthy variety of activities.

▶ *Can I ruck on a treadmill?*
Absolutely! Rucking outdoors on varied terrain engages stabilizer muscles, helps improve balance, and, combined with fresh air and changing scenery, boosts mental health and reduces boredom. But

when it's not practical or safe to ruck outside, indoor options can help you stay consistent. Rucking on a treadmill or stair climber offers an excellent alternative during inclement weather. (Rucking embraces the suck, though, so don't be afraid of the elements as long as you're not sacrificing safety.)

Treadmill rucking gives you total control of all variables: weight, incline, speed, and duration. Simulate hills by increasing the incline while maintaining a steady pace, or push your limits with interval training. The stair climber offers a more intense challenge, focusing on lower body strength by targeting legs and glutes, making it a great variation for building endurance and muscle simultaneously.

► *Can my kids ruck with me?*

You bet! Rucking is a wonderful way to share quality time as a family. Exploring local trails, walking to a nearby park, or just strolling the neighborhood sets a positive example for kids. Plus, they often love carrying an "adventure pack," and you can turn a ruck into a scavenger hunt, encouraging exploration along the way. Rucking as a family fosters healthy habits that can last a lifetime.

A couple of precautions and posture cues differentiate children from adults, though. Due to their center of gravity, kids may find it more comfortable to carry a pack lower on their back. To promote good posture and avoid forward head tilt, loads should never exceed 10 to 15 percent of a child's body weight.[26]

► *Will rucking make my back pain worse?*

Back pain has many origins, such as muscle imbalances, poor posture, or injury. Rucking may counteract some back pain by improving posture and strengthening muscles in the back, shoulders, and core. Check with your health provider first and, if you get the go-ahead, ease into it. To avoid inducing or exacerbating back pain, invest in a well-designed rucksack that distributes weight evenly across your back and shoulders. Begin with light weight and always maintain good form. Keep your shoulders back and engage your core to avoid leaning forward. Maintaining proper alignment reduces stress on the spine and encourages healthier movement.

Pay attention to your body. If pain develops, intensifies, or feels sharp, stop immediately and consult a healthcare professional.

### ▶ Will rucking help me lose weight?

Rucking increases calorie expenditure, which can help with weight loss. Additionally, gaining muscle increases metabolic rate, meaning you'll burn more calories at rest. As any athlete will tell you, though, a higher metabolism means increased appetite. Successful weight loss happens through nutrition because what you consume affects results more than how much you burn by rucking, walking, or training. Rucking reduces stress, which helps curb emotional eating, and it promotes better sleep, which plays a critical role in blood sugar management and appetite regulation. Remember, you can't out-ruck a bad diet; your diet does the heavy lifting when it comes to creating the calorie deficit needed to lose weight.

### ▶ Can I use a weighted vest?

Yes. Rucking traditionally involves carrying a weighted backpack, but a weighted vest works just fine, too. Both options have advantages, and choosing the right one depends on your goals, comfort, and preferences.

A weighted vest, for example, distributes weight evenly across the torso, which can feel more stable, but it may not yield the same posture improvements as a rucksack. While less bulky, a weighted vest can trap heat and restrict breathing, which might lead to discomfort, particularly in hot or humid conditions. Weighted vests often come in fixed weight increments, meaning you likely will need to buy a vest at a specific weight.

Rucksacks, on the other hand, offer more flexibility. You can easily add or remove weight plates or other heavy items, making it a better option for beginners who may be scaling up quickly. Rucksacks provide more versatility, storage capacity, and physiological benefits, such as improved breathing mechanics and postural alignment.

Test both options to see which feels more comfortable and suits your goals. See Chapter 3 for more on gear.

▶ *Is rucking better than running?*
It depends on your goals and preferences. Rucking is lower impact than running, making it easier on joints and a great option for beginners. Running, on the other hand, works better for anyone who is focused on high-intensity exercise or is looking to achieve a speed or race-specific goal. Compared to unweighted walking, rucking slightly increases the load on your knees, but still falls well below the impact of running.

Runners tend to experience a higher rate of injury, with common issues including shin splints, stress fractures, and runner's knee. These aches and pains come from the repetitive, high-impact nature of the activity, in which force exerted on the knees can equal up to *five* times your body weight with every stride. Rucking distributes weight more evenly and reduces joint stress, making it a safer alternative if you're concerned about knee health. Both activities require careful progression, stringent attention to form, and adequate recovery to minimize injury risk.

▶ *Which burns more calories, rucking or running?*
That varies based on body weight, terrain, pace, duration, and weight carried. Running generally burns more calories per minute, but the low-impact nature of rucking means people can ruck

for longer periods. The calorie burns look comparable. Both exercises require minimal equipment and allow you to take your workout outside. Each activity has its benefits. Rucking causes less wear and tear on the body, whereas running can improve speed and maximize cardiovascular fitness. Try both, see which aligns with your goals and lifestyle best, and incorporate them into your routine accordingly.

# PREVENTING INJURY

When you start, your body will adjust to carrying a ruck. Shoulder discomfort and muscle soreness are common, especially for beginners. Early on, I noticed an annoying pinch in my right shoulder that took four to six weeks to resolve. Minor discomfort is part of the process. With regular rucks, your body will adapt to the extra load.

Not to be overlooked, footwear is another important piece of the puzzle. The first few times I rucked, I noticed my usual walking shoes didn't offer enough support, which led to discomfort, especially after long rucks. A stiffer boot provided the stability I needed and made a world of difference. Before strapping on extra weight, gradually increase time on your feet. Keep your feet dry and avoid friction within the shoe. More on choosing the right footwear in Chapter 3.

## *Discomfort versus Pain*

As you start rucking, it's crucial to understand the difference between discomfort and pain. Discomfort might feel like a dull, tired sensation in your muscles or a nagging pinch, like in my shoulder. Physical cues like this are expected and indicate your body is working and adapting.

Pain, however, feels different. Sharp, persistent, or alarming sensations can signal overexertion or injury. Pain can present as tingling, numbness, or unusual discomfort in joints or nerves. If you feel pain, especially in your joints or tingling or numbness elsewhere, *stop*. If you're mid-ruck, adjust your pack or reduce the weight.

Rucksack palsy can occur when the weight of a backpack compresses nerves in the shoulder, leading to weakness, numbness, or even temporary paralysis of the arm. This can happen if your ruck is too heavy, worn incorrectly, or carried for long periods without making adjustments. Rucksack palsy usually happens with military personnel carrying up to half of their body weight, so it's not common for civilians—but it can happen. If you develop persistent pain or tingling, consult a professional.

To mitigate shoulder discomfort and avoid injury, try one or more of the following techniques:

**Use the right pack.** Your ruck should fit snugly but not feel too restrictive. Carry the weight high and tight. For larger packs or heavier loads, rest the weight on your hips, not your shoulders.

**Adjust straps for maximum comfort.** Shift the weight and cinch pack straps as needed, so you can stretch your shoulders and arms to maintain good circulation and reduce nerve compression.

**Avoid excessively heavy loads.** Begin light and gradually increase the weight as your body adapts.

**Use bubble wrap or a towel as filler to secure and cushion the load.** You want the weight sturdy and stable in your pack and snug against your back.

**Pay attention to posture.** If you're slouching forward, the weight is too heavy. Engage your core and glutes. Press your hips forward, shoulder blades down and back, and release unnecessary tension in your neck and jaw.

**Go slow and steady.** It's not a race. Take short, strong strides.

# ADVANCED STRATEGIES

Growth happens when you push yourself outside your comfort zone. To reap the full benefits, rucking has to suck enough, which means you'll encounter your fair share of discomfort. Once you've mastered the basic mechanics, you can manipulate three key variables—weight, speed, and incline—to increase the intensity of your rucks.

In strength and endurance training, progressive overload involves gradually increasing difficulty over time. Systematically introducing new challenges forces the body to adapt, building strength, endurance, and all-around fitness. Here's why progressive overload is worth the extra effort:

**Break through plateaus.** Increasing the difficulty of your workouts sets you up for consistent improvement.

**Personalize your progress.** Whether you're a beginner looking to find your base weight or a seasoned rucker tackling rugged terrain, you can customize a training plan to your unique needs.

**Minimize injury risk.** Gradual adaptation reduces the likelihood of overtraining, which helps avoid injury and minimize mental burnout.

**Enhance resilience.** Overcoming progressively harder challenges builds grit. Each successful ruck reinforces mental and physical perseverance.

**Prevent boredom.** Varying weight, speed, and terrain keeps your workouts fresh and engaging. Variety in your training routine helps keep you motivated.

No one-size-fits-all training strategy exists. Every approach, including progressive overload, has potential drawbacks. For instance, pushing too hard with heavier weight or on challenging terrain, without adequate rest and recovery, can lead to fatigue, soreness, and diminishing returns. Strength and endurance take time to build, and overreaching too quickly often leads to burnout or injury. Progress isn't always linear, and results aren't always immediate, but consistency and patience do pay off.

Let's explore how to use weight, speed, and incline to make your rucks more productive with just the right amount of suck. But remember to change only *one* variable at a time to help avoid injury.

## *Increase the Weight*

Carrying a heavier load forces your body to adapt by using more muscle and demanding higher cardiovascular output, resulting in increased strength and endurance. Start with a manageable weight that feels challenging but doesn't overtax your body. Once you establish your base weight, stick with it for at least two to four weeks, then increase the load in 10 percent increments. Yes, that could mean adding just 2 or 3 pounds at a time. If you finish a ruck and forget about the weight entirely, that's one sign you're ready for more. Slowly build your ruck weight until you reach no more than 25 to 30 percent of your body weight. Not everyone will reach this threshold. I certainly haven't yet!

In the beginning, I used a 10-pound ruck plate, which felt easy and caused only a few harmless cricks and creaks from the change in posture and gait. After three weeks, I added 5 pounds and rucked with 15 pounds for three to four weeks before adding another 5 pounds. It took nearly two months to go from 10 pounds to 20 pounds, and no two days felt the same. Some felt easy, and other rucks felt hard—all of which is 100 percent normal.

To increase training volume or total workload, consider incorporating strength exercises before, during, or after a ruck. If you want to maximize muscle, especially in your lower body, add squats, lunges, or step-ups to your routine. For instance, incorporate 5 to 20 squats or lunges throughout your ruck or sandwich it with strength moves. For more simple hacks, see Chapter 4.

## Pick Up the Pace

Rucking faster increases cardiovascular demand, boosts endurance, and provides an easily trackable metric for progress. But first, you have to know your baseline. To find your pace, clock your ruck with a timer or fitness tracker. Stick to a specific distance: once around the block, 1 mile, or 2 miles. With this information, you can calculate an average pace—a 20-minute mile, for example. After that, gradually increase your speed and reduce your time. If you like to listen to music while you ruck, playlists that focus on beats per minute (bpm) make this strategy a breeze. The more beats per minute, the faster you'll go. For many ruckers, a goal of 15 to 20 minutes per mile strikes a sweet spot between challenge and sustainability. Gently push yourself to walk faster while maintaining good form and control of the weight.

Another method for pushing tempo is to incorporate speed intervals. Warm up for 5 to 10 minutes, then push into a near-jog or "ruck shuffle" for bursts of 30 to 60 seconds before returning to your usual pace. A ruck shuffle splits the difference between a fast walk and a jog. Keep your feet close to the ground, taking quick, short strides. Pump your arms to help drive your momentum forward and maintain a steady rhythm. Ruck shuffling works great if you want to increase your cardiovascular fitness and stamina without the impact of running. Never run while wearing weight, though. Ruck *or* run, but never both at the same time.

Remember, not every ruck is a race. Give yourself slower-paced days to enjoy the journey, avoid burnout, and keep it fun.

## Change the Terrain

After you've built a solid base with weight and speed on flat terrain, you can up the difficulty by increasing the incline. Adding elevation is the most effective way to take your rucks to the next level. Just a 1 percent increase in grade demands *10 times* more energy than a 1 percent increase in weight.[27] That boost costs nothing except a little legwork to find a nearby slope or hill. The steeper the incline, the greater the gains.

Rucking downhill is also important for balance, coordination, and stability, helping you feel sure-footed and avoiding fall-related injuries. After you've mastered inclines and declines, head to trails with uneven ground. For example, rucking on sand or snow uses muscles you didn't even know you had. These kinds of terrains create natural resistance, demanding extra effort from your body. For winter rucking, always wear proper footwear, such as ice cleats and thermal gear, and exercise caution.

Apps such as AllTrails or Strava allow you to view the difficulty, distance, and elevation change of local trails and scout new locations. If you're stuck indoors, ruck on a treadmill, which gives you total control of speed and incline. Don't hold the handrails or console, though. Holding on to the machine counteracts the incline, which defeats the purpose! If you don't feel steady rucking on a treadmill, reduce the speed until you can tolerate the incline without holding on to anything. For added security, use the safety key or clip, which will stop the machine immediately if you fall or move too far away from the controls.

Regardless of how you choose to ramp up your ruck, never change more than one variable at a time. If you're rucking a new trail, for instance, consider lowering your ruck weight and/or slowing down to avoid injury. Like seasoning in a recipe, ruck to your taste and adjust each component—weight, speed, incline—until you've crafted a recipe that suits your goal.

# REST AND RECOVERY

Gains don't happen during exercise; they happen during recovery. Without adequate rest, physical stress can shift from a positive stimulus for growth to a setback. Instead of getting stronger, your body might show signs of muscle breakdown, fatigue, and declining performance. Some stress benefits physical fitness, sure, but chronic stress increases cortisol levels, which, if unchecked, can weaken your immune system, degrade sleep, and disrupt recovery. Worse yet, overtraining and improper recovery can lead to injury that might sideline you for weeks or even months. Make time to rest, repair, and rebuild through quality sleep, good nutrition, and active recovery—or your body will do it for you.

Many people struggle with this step. If you have a driven, all-or-nothing mindset, even just the *idea* of slowing down can feel counterproductive, even lazy. But recovery is a strategic, scientific tool—not a sign of weakness. On the flip side, some people use rest as an excuse to slack off or skip workouts altogether, turning recovery into a permission slip to avoid doing the work. As with any long-term goal, you need to be intentional about what you're doing. Too little stress, and you won't make progress. Push too hard without sufficient rest, and you risk undermining your progress. Use the Goldilocks principle to find a balance between stress and rest that feels right to you: not too little, not too much—*just* enough.

With rucking, more risk lies in overdoing it, so let's look at common signs of overtraining or inadequate recovery.

### Physical
Persistent muscle soreness or stiffness.
Frequent injuries, such as strains, sprains, or stress fractures.
Elevated resting heart rate or feeling unusually depleted after a workout.

### Performance
Low motivation to train or feeling burned out.
Notable decline in training metrics.
Plateaus or regression in ability, despite consistent effort.

### Sleep and Immune System
Trouble falling or staying asleep, even when physically exhausted.
Getting sick more often, such as frequent colds or other infections.

### Mental and Emotional
Chronic fatigue or exhaustion that doesn't improve with sleep.
Difficulty concentrating or lack of mental clarity (brain fog).
Increased irritability, mood swings, or feelings of depression.
Lack of interest in activities that you typically enjoy.

If you recognize more than a couple of these symptoms, step back and prioritize rest and recovery. Doing so will help reduce cortisol, the hormone responsible for many of the symptoms listed above. Some cortisol is normal, but too much can increase muscle breakdown and accelerate fat storage—a double-whammy against all your hard work.

Focus on stress relief rather than chasing personal bests. During periods of high psychological stress, literally lighten the load to reduce physical strain and prioritize time spent outside to boost mood and mental clarity.

Recovery doesn't mean just sitting still, though. Strategic rest actively supports your body's ability to heal and rebuild. Intentional recovery practices can help you build stronger muscles, better endurance, and a more resilient self. Here are several ways to program active recovery into your daily or weekly routine:

**Move gently.** Low-intensity activities such as walking, stretching, yoga, or foam rolling keep blood flowing to your muscles, helping to decrease soreness, eliminate metabolic waste, and accelerate healing. Chapter 4 includes some feel-good stretches to complement your rucks.

**Embrace body work.** Massage therapy, chiropractic care, acupuncture, and other manual techniques help release muscle tension, improve blood flow, and speed recovery.

**Explore temperature therapy.** Alternating hot treatments for sore muscles and cold treatments for inflammation promote blood flow and relaxation. Soothe your body and unwind with a warm bath or sauna. After intense workouts, take an ice bath or cold shower to decompress and boost mental resilience.

**Eat well.** A healthy diet with a good balance of macronutrients—protein, healthy fats, and carbohydrates—is essential for muscle repair and energy replenishment. Focus on nutrient-dense, whole foods and stay hydrated to support your body's recovery. See Chapter 5 for more on nutrition.

**Get good sleep.** This is a nonnegotiable. Aim for seven to nine hours per night. Good sleep starts in the morning with direct sunlight, which helps keep your circadian rhythm on track. At night, a diligent wind-down routine helps prepare your mind and body for the rest it needs.

**Take rest days.** These full breaks from training give your muscles time to heal and regenerate. Think of rest days as an investment in your next workout. They create a necessary energy reservoir for the hard work that enables long-term gains in strength and stamina.

**Relieve stress.** Incorporate mindfulness practices such as meditation or deep breathing exercises to mitigate tension and promote mental resiliency.

Remember the Goldilocks rule to discover the right balance and listen to your body. In the long run, prioritizing recovery won't just keep you in the game—it makes you better at it.

## REMEMBER

► Start by walking, then transition to rucking with gear you already have.

► Begin with a light load and increase gradually, no more than 10 percent at a time.

► When you feel comfortable, increase weight, speed, and incline, but don't change more than one variable at a time.

► Listen to your body to avoid injuries from too much weight, incorrect posture, the wrong footwear, and overtraining.

► Practice intentional recovery techniques for maximum gains in strength and stamina.

# 3

# Gear and Gadgets

Take care of your gear, and your
gear will take care of you.

—JOCKO WILLINK,
AUTHOR AND RETIRED US NAVY SEAL

Rucking doesn't have to be expensive or complicated. Chances are, you already have what you need to begin. Start with a backpack, add some weight—books, canned goods, water bottles—and go for a walk. As you build strength and carry heavier loads, then you might consider buying reinforced or ruck-specific gear. It might seem like an unnecessary expense, but investing in quality equipment can save money by taking your workout outside and eliminating the need for a gym membership. Good gear helps you carry more weight more comfortably. It's a tangible way to invest in your health and while reinforcing your dedication to long-term fitness goals.

Even if you purchase gear, rucking is still one of the most cost-effective ways to get and stay fit. It doesn't come with monthly fees, crowded spaces, or limited hours. You can work out anywhere, and your ruck can serve as an all-in-one piece of fitness equipment, a

Swiss Army knife for exercise. Wear your ruck to boost cardiovascular endurance or use it in place of free weights to build strength (Chapter 4 covers ruck-specific strength movements). And quality rucking gear is built to last. Companies like GORUCK offer lifetime warranties on their rucksacks, so you can rest assured that your investment is well spent.

Many people customize their rucksacks with patches for added inspiration. Some badges include motivational quotes such as "Embrace the Suck," while others signify completing a difficult event or grueling mileage. My favorite patch quote comes from Sarah: "Just because someone carries it well, doesn't mean it isn't heavy." A few well-placed words or visual cues can remind you how far you've come or where you want to go in your fitness journey.

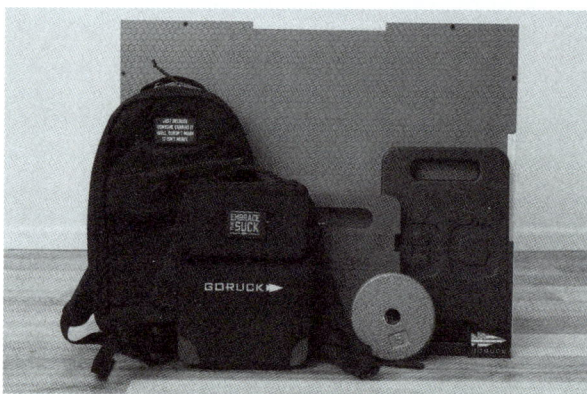

## PICKING YOUR PACK

Rucking isn't just about the weight you carry but also how you carry it. Backpack design plays a critical role in comfort and performance. It's important to consider ergonomics and how efficiently you can move while under load. Rucking shouldn't feel *easy*, but maintaining good posture and proficient movement helps maximize your workout while minimizing unnecessary strain.

As you increase the weight, pack design becomes increasingly important for injury prevention and comfort. A standard backpack will suffice for lighter loads, but more weight means being more deliberate with your gear. Heavier loads demand a durable pack with padded, sturdy shoulder straps and a hip belt to ensure good posture and effective load distribution. The right setup can make the difference between a successful ruck and a bad one. Let's look at the various options.

## Rucksacks versus Backpacks

A standard backpack may work for light loads, but it's not designed for heavy-duty weights. My husband and I learned this lesson the hard way. We cycled through several old backpacks and cheap hiking packs that failed the test of added tension and load. Stitching ripped, handles tore off, and cuss words flew. It wasn't pretty.

Bigger loads require a beefier setup. In a regular backpack, weight tends to sag, causing discomfort and distraction. A rucksack, however, is purpose-built for carrying heavy weight over long distances. With reinforced handles and stitching, it won't stretch or tear under heftier loads, and it features padded shoulder straps for extra comfort. The design holds the weight higher and closer to the back for maximum efficiency and weight distribution.

For extra support, choose a rucksack with a sternum or chest strap in addition to a hip belt. A hip belt significantly lowers the rate of perceived exertion, a subjective measure of physical effort, which means your ruck feels easier even when the load stays the same.[28] Women should consider the location and adjustability of the chest strap. The strap can feel quite uncomfortable if it falls across the bustline and can't be moved. Always test your ruck before heading out, as the load can shift and affect strap positioning.

The combination of a hip belt and chest strap allows you to cinch the load closer to your body and spread the weight to different muscle groups. For example, you can leverage upper body strength by tightening the chest strap. To distribute weight to your hips, tighten the belt to your midsection and loosen the upper body strap. This flexibility enhances comfort, enabling you to ruck longer, heavier, and harder.

Rucksacks also have dedicated pockets for weight plates, making it easy to swap and customize the load. A quality rucksack can handle loads up to 30 percent of your body weight, making it the most versatile choice for serious rucking.

**Pros:** No weight limit, ample storage, adjustable padded straps

**Cons:** Bulkier than other options

**Best for:** A durable, versatile, no-limitation option

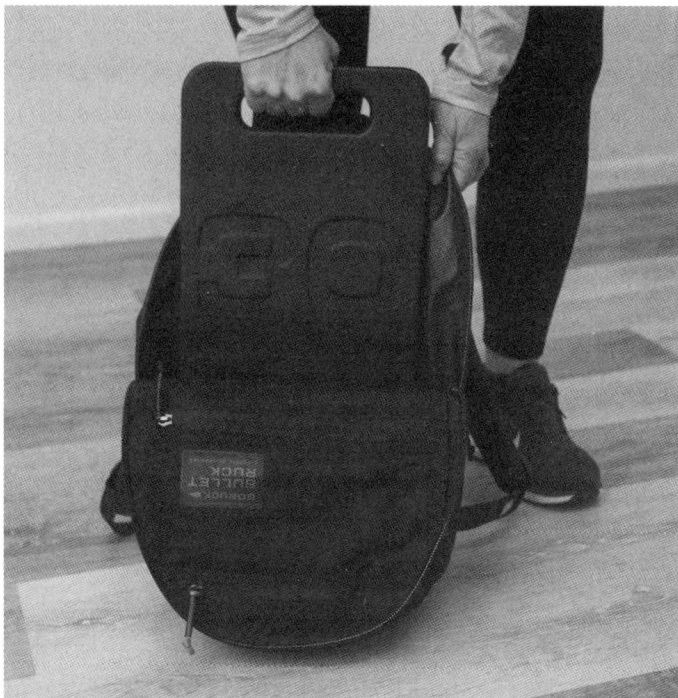

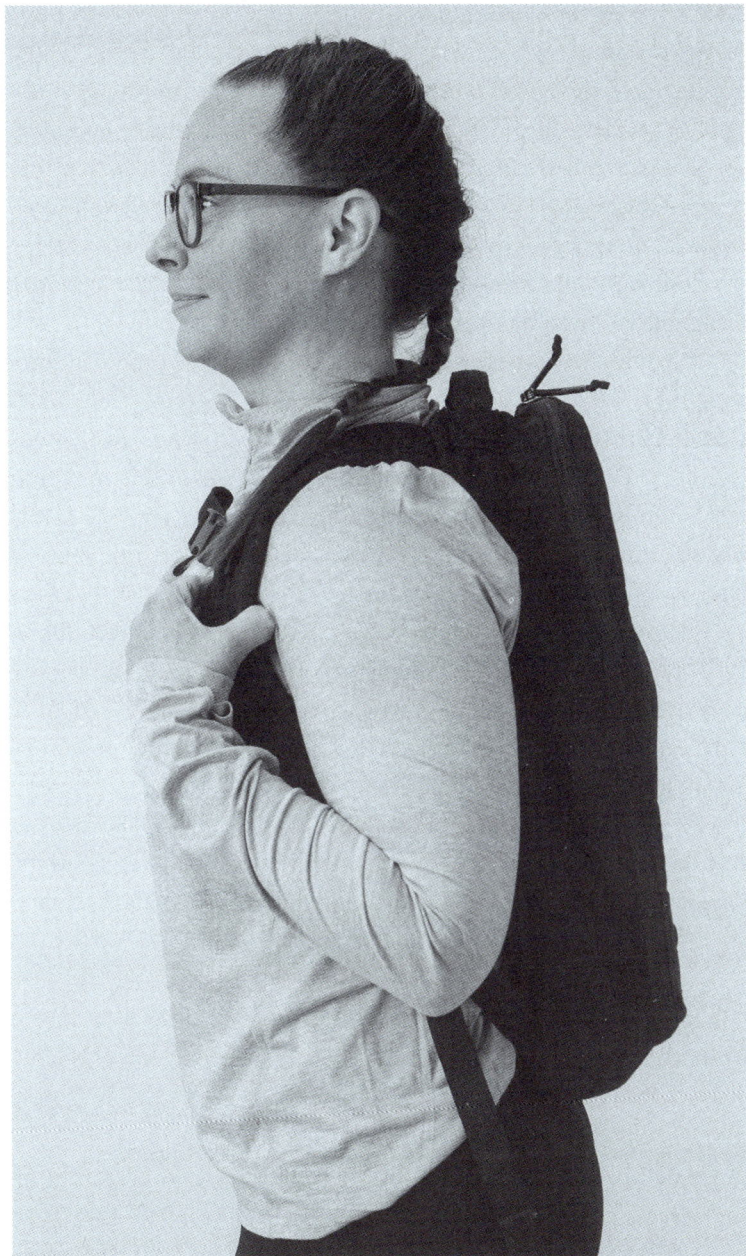

## Ruck Plate Carriers

Abbreviated RPC, this minimalist alternative to a rucksack holds one or two weight plates. It contains no extra storage compartment, which is a drawback for longer rucks that require water and snacks. But the low-profile design makes it ideal for neighborhood walks, gym sessions, or adding resistance to everyday movement.

Compact and efficient, RPCs have their limitations. Most are designed for no more than 30 or 45 pounds, so if you want to ruck heavier than that, opt for a rucksack. RPCs have one pocket for a weight plate, but not all weight plates will fit. Measure the pocket dimensions to ensure that your plate fits. Body shape also comes into play. People with broad shoulders or larger builds may find RPCs too tight in the upper arm and armpit areas. RPCs rarely include hip belts, which means they don't offer the same level of load distribution.

People either love RPCs or hate them. I own a rucksack and an RPC, both from GORUCK, and I personally love my RPC. It's my go-to for shorter rucks and grab-and-go workouts. The GORUCK RPC is available in standard and long, the latter suited for taller people, those with thicker frames, or anyone wanting to carry the 45-pound RPC limit. For rucks around the neighborhood, the standard RPC works great for me, and a rucksack makes sense for longer rucks where I pack water and day-hike essentials.

**Pros:** Less expensive than a rucksack, compact, sturdy for light-to-moderate weights

**Cons:** Limited weight capacity, no extra storage, challenging for broader builds

**Best for:** A minimalist, lightweight, streamlined option

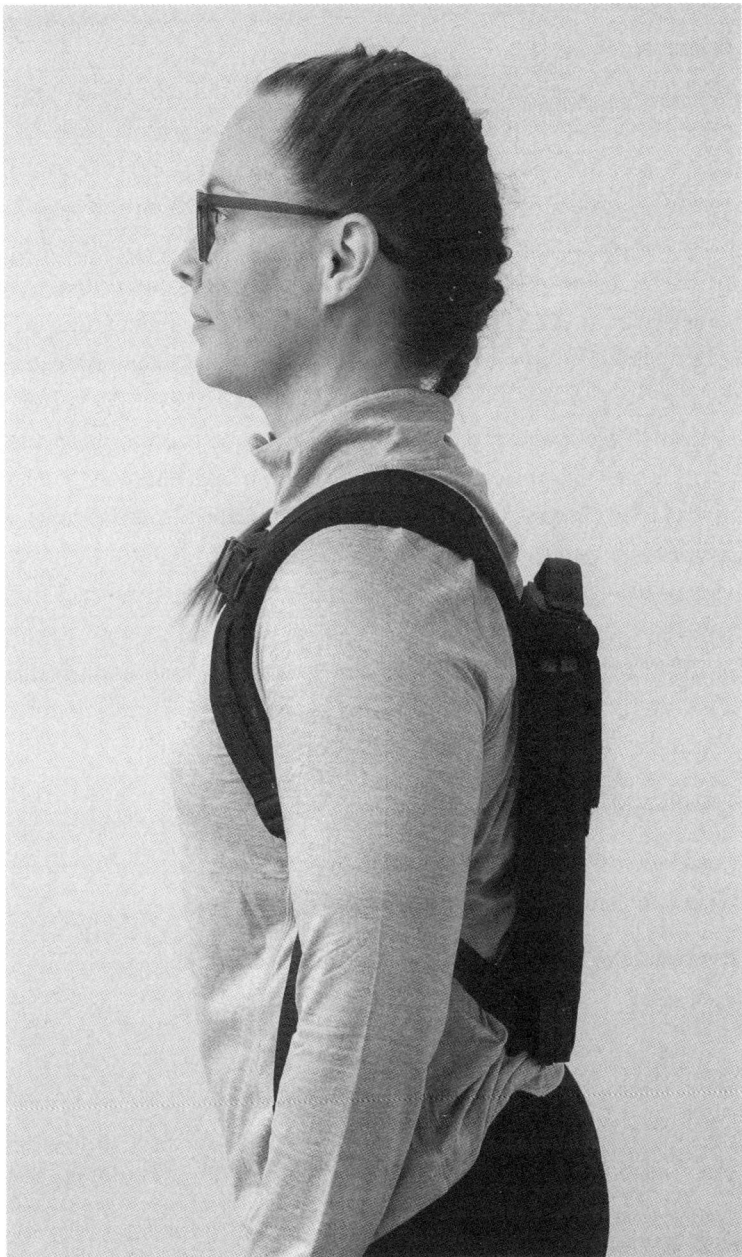

## Weighted Vests

Like RPCs, weighted vests are another minimalist option. Vests often come at a fixed weight, so they offer less customization. You may be able to find options that allow you to insert or remove small weights to adjust the load without purchasing a whole new vest.

Vests make a great option for workouts, but they differ significantly from rucksacks in how they impact your posture. A weighted vest distributes the load evenly across the front and back. This compresses the spine, and you can't lean into the weight like you can with a rucksack. Vests can also affect breathing and heat dissipation. Full-body styles covering the chest may restrict lung expansion, particularly during high-intensity rucks. In warm or humid weather, they can trap heat against the body, a problem for people who run hot. To mitigate these issues, choose a vest with weight distributed throughout the straps and back, not over the chest.

Weighted vests work best for lightweight, short-duration activities or for people who need extra stability. For long-distance rucking or heavy loads, stick with a rucksack.

**Pros:** Stable, evenly distributed weight

**Cons:** Potentially restrict breathing and trap heat against the body, limited scalability, less beneficial for posture

**Best for:** Stability or a simple, fixed-weight option

► ► ►

When selecting a carrying system, consider your goals, typical rucking conditions, and comfort preferences. It's not a fashion show, so get started with what you've got, and upgrade as your needs evolve. Remember these tips to make the most of whichever pack you choose.

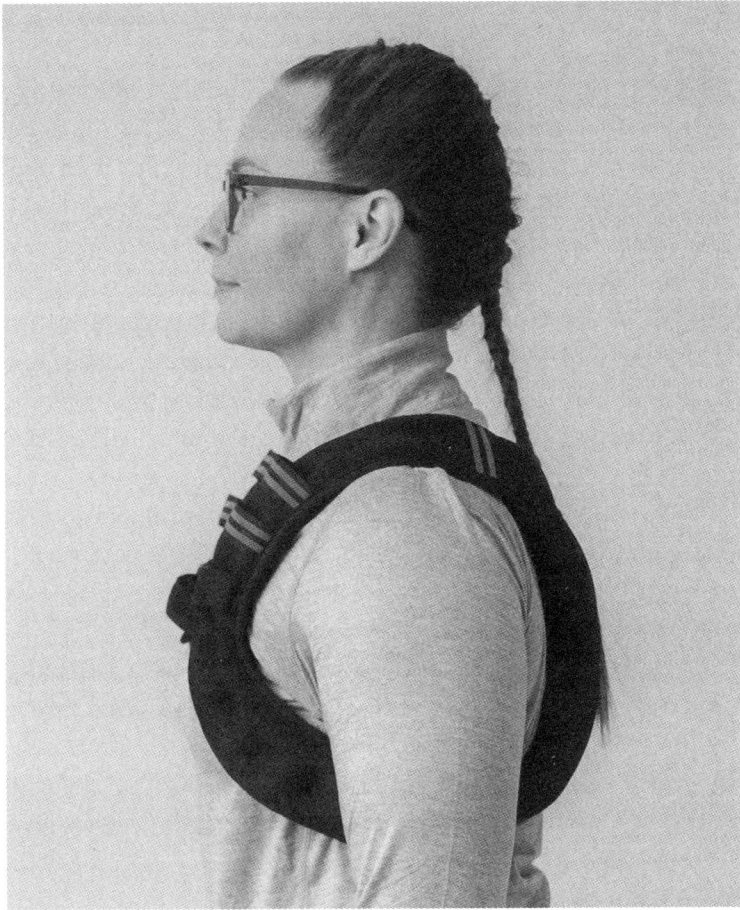

- Opt for padded, adjustable shoulder straps.
- Fasten the weight high and tight on your back.
- Always use both shoulder straps.
- Cinch straps, so they feel snug but not too restrictive.
- Use a hip belt for heavier loads.
- In hot, humid weather, choose a carrying system that doesn't position weight over your chest.

# WEIGHTS AND PLATES

After you choose your pack, it's time to focus on the weight. The type of weight you use and how you position it will determine the comfort and effectiveness of your ruck. You can ruck with anything heavy, but bulky objects and odd shapes can make for an awkward or uncomfortable fit. By design, ruck plates are the most suitable fit in a rucksack or backpack pocket. Most ruck plates have a compact, flat, rectangular design, so they sit flush against your back, minimizing movement and maximizing weight distribution. Often, they're made of cast iron with a powder coat to prevent rusting, which is especially useful if you live in a humid climate or ruck in damp conditions.

Before purchasing ruck plates, measure the dimensions of your backpack pocket or rucksack's plate compartment. A snug fit ensures the plate remains stable while you move, improving your comfortability and concentration during a ruck.

Start with lighter plates and increase the weight gradually. Look for a system that allows you to add or swap plates easily. For example, instead of purchasing one 20-pound ruck plate, opt for two 10-pound plates or one 10-pound plate and two 5-pound plates. This arrangement gives you more flexibility to increase or decrease the load if you want to toy with other variables such as speed and incline.

Always use the internal pocket in a rucksack or backpack to keep the weight stable and close to your body. If you ruck with more than one weight plate, it can help to tether plates together with tape or a strap. You can also pad plates with a towel or bubble wrap to prevent them from clanking against one another and secure them in your pack.

# FOOTWEAR AND FOOT CARE

The right shoes or boots protect your feet, align your posture, and set the foundation for a good ruck. Wearing the wrong footwear can lead to discomfort, blisters, foot fatigue, plantar fasciitis, shin splints, and other painful conditions. Your choice of footwear depends heavily on the terrain, weather, and personal preference. Some ruckers swear by hiking boots for added ankle support and durability, especially on uneven or rugged trails. Others prefer lightweight, low-profile options such as trail runners or tennis shoes, which can provide added agility and comfort on smoother surfaces. There's no one-size-fits-all *sole*-ution (not sorry) for footwear. It may take some trial and error to discover what works best for you. Your ideal rucking footwear should be:

**Sturdy and supportive.** The shoe or boot needs to provide adequate internal padding to absorb the impact of walking with weight. If needed, consider inserts for extra cushioning or arch support, but avoid too much squish.

**Traction focused.** Rubber soles with good grip work well for diverse terrains, especially uneven or slippery surfaces.

**Comfortable.** A secure fit around the heel prevents blisters, while a wide toe box keeps your toes from pinching on descents.

**Environmentally appropriate.** Breathable materials help your feet stay dry and comfortable. Waterproof shoes keep water out, but they also trap moisture in; so know your feet and your terrain.

On longer rucks, foot fatigue, blisters, and chafing can escalate quickly. Good foot hygiene and proper attire, including high-quality socks, keep your feet dry, comfortable, and blister-free. As former Green Beret Jason McCarthy says, socks are "life and death" for soldiers. If you plan to ruck through tough terrain, don't take his wisdom as an exaggeration. He spent *two years* finding the right sock supplier for GORUCK. Socks are that important, so invest in good, moisture-wicking material.

After long rucks, give your feet a good look over for hot spots—areas of redness, warmth, or irritation—which are precursors to painful blisters. Early identification and prevention are key: If you notice a hot spot that hasn't developed into a blister, consider covering the area with athletic tape or a blister bandage for added protection. If a blister does form, gently pierce and drain it while leaving the top layer of skin intact. Dab it with antibiotic ointment, cover it with a sterile bandage, and put on dry socks. When you're done rucking, let your feet air out and give the blister time to dry, which can speed the healing process and get you back on your feet.

Be proactive and follow these foot-care tips:

**Trim your toenails.** Keep toenails clipped to avoid unnecessary pressure and help prevent ingrown nails.

**Don't skimp on socks.** Moisture-wicking socks made of wool or synthetic fibers help keep feet dry and reduce friction. Cotton socks trap moisture and increase the risk of blisters, so avoid those. Never wear more than one pair of socks. Instead, try socks with different thicknesses, and change into a dry pair if they get damp.

**Break in footwear first.** Never tackle long distances with new shoes or boots. Gradually break them in on shorter walks, giving your feet time to adjust.

# EXTRAS

A few thoughtful extras can make your rucking experience safer, more comfortable, and more enjoyable. If you're traveling unfamiliar trails, rugged terrain, or a desolate area, carrying some or all the following items in your rucksack is worthwhile. Depending on the environment and length of the ruck, consider bringing:

**First aid kit:** A good, compact kit should include bandages of a few different sizes, antiseptic wipes, antibiotic ointment, and any medications you may need.

**Bug spray:** On wooded trails especially, bug spray fends off mosquitoes, ticks, and other insects. For maximum protection, look for options with DEET or, if you prefer going chemical-free, choose a natural alternative. For long-lasting bug protection, spray your gear with permethrin, which can last up to 6 weeks.

**Hydration:** For longer rucks, consider a hydration bladder, so you can sip without stopping. Know your refill spots and, if needed, bring a portable filtration device. For hot or sweaty rucks, electrolyte supplements replenish lost minerals. See more on fluids and electrolytes in Chapter 5.

**Food:** Pack shelf-stable, portable, nutritious snacks such as protein bars, tuna packets with crackers, and trail mix. Bring a bag for trash so you can pack out what you pack in; leave no trace.

**Extra socks:** Wet feet are a rucker's worst nightmare. Bring an extra pair of moisture-wicking socks in case your feet get wet or sweaty.

**Trekking poles:** For rucks on uneven terrain, steep trails, or long distances, trekking poles can help with balance and posture. Telescoping options allow for easy stowing, when you're not using them.

# CLOTHING

Some materials wear better than others. Carrying a rucksack or weighted vest can interfere with heat dissipation, so moisture-wicking clothing will help you stay cool and dry. For the base layer, which is closest to your skin, opt for polyester, nylon, wool, and other fabrics that draw sweat away from your body. This allows for quick evaporation and helps regulate your body temperature, making you less likely to overheat. In cold temperatures, a moisture-wicking base helps keep sweat off your skin and prevents the chills. Avoid cotton, which retains moisture.

Also consider these additional recommendations:

**Mid-layer:** In colder weather, pair a lightweight fleece or insulated jacket with your base layer. It should be breathable and easy to remove if you get too warm.

**Outer layer:** For rain or strong wind, choose a waterproof and wind-resistant jacket. When conditions are unpredictable, bring lightweight options you can easily tie around your waist or stow in your rucksack.

**Reflective gear:** If you ruck in the early morning, late evening, or on busy roads, a reflective vest, armbands, or pack strips can make you more visible to drivers. Don't forget a headlamp or clip-on light to illuminate your path.

**Hat or cap:** Choose headwear that protects you from the sun or inclement conditions and helps you stay warm in colder weather.

Experiment with different equipment strategies and adapt your gear to the task at hand. For example, Beth wears her RPC *under* her winter coat in cold weather. She also dons her RPC while doing house chores, while Sarah ruck-mows her lawn to make the most of each step. The key is to get creative with how and when you ruck, because the best gear is the kind you'll actually use.

## RUCKING ON A BUDGET

Gearing up for rucking doesn't have to strain your wallet. With some creativity and ingenuity, you can ruck comfortably and cost-effectively without any fancy equipment. If you're on a budget, use what you already have: an old backpack, books, water bottles, sealed bags of rice, even loose bricks. To source what you don't have, thrift stores can be a goldmine for inexpensive gear, although it might take some extra MacGyvering to achieve maximum comfort on a minimal budget.

To help you ruck comfortably and affordably, consider these practical, budget-friendly hacks:

**DIY weight plates.** Source loose bricks or small pavers instead of pricey metal weight plates. Cover them in duct tape, bubble wrap, or padding to prevent them from crumbling or shifting inside your bag.

**Cushion the load.** Wrap your weights in an old towel, throw blanket, or yoga mat to soften sharp edges and protect your back and shoulders.

**Support your pack's weight.** If your backpack doesn't have a laptop slot or interior pocket to stow the weight, you can create a makeshift padding system to secure the load. Use a yoga block, towel, or blanket to pad the bottom of your pack. Pool noodles work great as a bumper for sharp edges or to fill the bottom of the bag.

**Elevate the weight.** Many hiking backpacks include a hook for a hydration bladder. Use the hook to suspend the weight higher in the pack, so it doesn't rest on your lower back.

You can ruck almost anywhere for free. Explore your neighborhood, local parks, or nearby trails to keep your routine fun and interesting. Download a free hiking or rucking app such as AllTrails, Strava, or RuckWell to discover new routes and track your mileage.

At the end of the day, don't overthink it or let cost be an excuse not to start. "Just get out there and do it," says Beth. "I gave way more thought than I needed to the mechanics of strapping the weight on. You don't need to buy anything crazy. Start by filling up some water bottles and put them in a backpack." Water bottles work great because if the weight feels too heavy, you can drink or pour out the water until it feels right. Start simple, but most importantly, just *start*.

## REMEMBER

▶ Rucking is an accessible, cost-effective activity. Begin with basic household items, such as an old backpack and makeshift weights. As you progress, upgrade to purpose-built gear, including a rucksack and ruck plates.

▶ Each carrying system has benefits and limitations. A rucksack provides the most versatility, while a ruck plate carrier or weighted vest is a streamlined alternative. Consider your goals and preferences to find the right fit for you.

▶ Your feet are the foundation for a safe, comfortable ruck. Sturdy shoes and climate-appropiate clothing can make or break a ruck. Prioritize footwear and care, because every steps counts!

# 4

## Training Plans and Exercises

A good plan implemented today is better than
a perfect plan implemented tomorrow.

—GEORGE PATTON III,
US ARMY GENERAL

Rucking helps you build strength and endurance, but it's not an all-in-one solution. To maximize your results and stay injury-free, you need a well-rounded routine that incorporates strength and mobility exercises. Think of it like a meal. Rucking is the main course, while mobility work and strength training are side dishes. These additions complement performance, elevate overall fitness, and build confidence.

This chapter will guide you toward achieving a supermedium, *Ruck Fit* physique: not too big, not too small, strong yet agile, and metabolically resilient. It's not about quick fixes or shortcuts, though. It's about consistent effort and smart training. Whether you're brand-new to exercise or a seasoned gym rat looking to shake up your regimen, there's a plan here for you. These structured training plans bring everything together in a simple, progressive schedule. They meet you where you are, no gym membership or fancy equipment required.

But the most important part of any exercise journey is starting. It's easy to fall into an endless cycle of research and procrastination, looking for the "perfect" plan or waiting for the "right" time to begin. As author Gretchen Rubin said in *Better Than Before*, "Don't get it perfect, get it going." Some people thrive on structure, whereas others flourish with freedom and flexibility. Rucking works for either camp. You know you best, so if you prefer to freestyle, grab your ruck and get out there. If you find comfort in having a methodical plan, pick a program and put it into action.

# TRAINING PRINCIPLES

Three training principles—rucking, strength, and mobility—form the foundation of the *Ruck Fit* workout plans. Rucking, as the core of each program, builds aerobic fitness while encouraging muscle adaptation. Rucking can't replace resistance training, though, so strength days do the heavy lifting (pun intended). Mobility work is the final ingredient that brings everything together, keeping joints flexible and supporting a full range of motion. As a whole, these elements create a well-rounded fitness regimen that you can adapt to your schedule and ability.

As with any new training plan, ease into it. Avoid jumping in headfirst, and if you're starting from scratch, take the rest days. Your body will need an adjustment period and may feel sore from rucking alone. Once you've built a solid endurance base and feel more confident, layer in mobility exercises to improve flexibility and help prevent injuries. Finally, when you're ready, add strength training to round out your routine.

Strength training, resistance training, and (weight) lifting are interchangeable terms that involve challenging your muscles in new ways to enhance strength and boost metabolic health. No matter what you call it or what equipment you use—resistance bands, free weights, body weight, or your ruck—strength training is a skill that takes practice. Similar to rucking, refine your technique first, then increase weight and training volume over time, not all at once. Gradual progression ensures sustainable results without provoking injury.

If you're new to strength training, the learning curve can feel steep, but don't let it intimidate you. It can be as simple as a bodyweight lunge or as advanced as a freestanding barbell squat. If you're not sure where to begin, start light and easy. If you already know what you're doing and want to develop your own routines, go for it. As Peloton instructor Denis Morton says, "I make suggestions, you make decisions."

## THE RIGHT PLAN FOR YOU

Put your ego aside and follow your body's lead, especially in the early days of a new program. It takes personal awareness to know how much weight to use and when enough is enough. Don't forget the Goldilocks principle of fitness: finding a weight and plan that aren't too easy or too hard, but just right. Choose a training plan that pushes you out of your comfort zone, but not so far that you feel discouraged and quit.

**5K Training Program:** If you're relatively sedentary (fewer than 5,000 steps daily) or don't follow a structured workout routine, this plan is a great starting point. It also works well if you have limited time since the shorter distances fit easily into a busy schedule.

**10K Training Program:** For a greater challenge and longer distances, this plan offers more mileage while keeping flexibility top of mind. It's ideal if you have some exercise experience and are ready to build endurance and go the extra mile.

**Half-Marathon or 25K Training Program:** If you really want to push your limits and tackle a long-distance challenge, this plan is for you. A program of this caliber requires more time and effort, with some rucks lasting two to four hours, depending on your pace. It can prove physically taxing on your body, requiring adequate recovery. Complete the 10K plan before embarking on this program.

► ► ►

There's no one-size-fits-all rulebook, so feel free to adapt the plans to meet your needs. With any of them, you can increase or decrease the difficulty by modifying ruck weight, pace, and/or elevation. It can feel tempting to go all-in, but it's always better to start small. Finishing a session and feeling like you could have done more is better than overdoing it and throwing in the towel. If you can't decide between 5K or 10K, do the 5K first. You can always upgrade to the 10K later.

## *Events Boost Motivation*

For added motivation, consider signing up for a local 5K or 10K race that takes place near the end of your training program. You can turn any walking event into a rucking event—no special race required. Rucking with others or entering a race can help you stay accountable and consistent. Even if you don't enter to win, you can support a good cause and get a great workout, which makes for a win-win.

Avoid race-day mistakes such as wearing brand-new shoes, a fresh T-shirt, or other untested gear. Stick to what you already know. Also, use familiar fueling and hydration strategies. Race day isn't the time to experiment. If you sign up for a rucking event, research the course and know whether the race has a minimum weight requirement, such as the Norwegian Foot March (for more on the NFM, see A Brief History of Rucking on page 6). Some ruck events offer light, standard, and heavy options, depending on how much weight you want to carry. These weights often exclude water or other consumables. Read the event rules carefully to avoid any race-day surprises.

# 5K TRAINING PROGRAM

This beginner-friendly plan will take you from zero to 5K (3.1 miles) in eight weeks. It applies progressive overload by increasing weight, distance, and intensity gradually to ensure safe, sustainable results. Each week focuses on specific goals, such as practicing proper posture and experimenting with variable speeds and terrain. By the end, you'll have completed your first 5K ruck and should feel stronger, leaner, and more confident.

## Overview

| Week | Rucks per Week | Duration | Distance | Weight | Focus |
|------|------|----------|----------|--------|-------|
| 1 | 2 or 3 | 20–30 minutes | 1 mile | 5–15 pounds | posture, walking under load |
| 2 | 3 | 30 minutes | 1.5 miles | 10–15 pounds | increased pace and distance |
| 3 | 3 | 30–40 minutes | 1.5 miles | 10–15 pounds | slight hills or varied terrain for 1 ruck |
| 4 | 3 | 30–40 minutes | 2 miles | 10–20 pounds | 15–20 minutes per mile for 1 ruck |
| 5 | 3 | 40–50 minutes | 2.5 miles | 10–20 pounds | plus 10–15 minutes strength exercises after 1 ruck |
| 6 | 3 or 4 | 40–50 minutes | 2.5 miles | 15–30 pounds | steeper terrain for 1 ruck |
| 7 | 3 or 4 | 50 minutes–1 hour | 3 miles | 15–30 pounds | pacing the full 5K |
| 8 | 2 or 3 | 50 minutes | 3 miles | 15–30 pounds | reserve energy to complete the 5K |

## Sample Workout Calendar

This schedule balances rucking with strength training, mobility work, and optional rest days to ensure that you're building strength and endurance while minimizing the risk of injury. Feel free to adjust the days to fit your weekly routine but aim to maintain the structure of rucking plus optional cross-training to optimize recovery and progress.

| Day | Weeks 1–4 | Weeks 5–8 |
| --- | --- | --- |
| Monday | strength training or rest | strength training or rest |
| Tuesday | regular ruck, 20–40 minutes | regular ruck, 40 minutes–1 hour |
| Wednesday | mobility work or rest | mobility work or rest |
| Thursday | regular ruck, 20–40 minutes | lightweight ruck, 40 minutes–1 hour |
| Friday | strength training or rest | strength training or rest |
| Saturday | long ruck, 1–2 miles | long ruck, 2.5–3.1 miles |
| Sunday | mobility work or rest | mobility work or rest |

## Components

**Regular rucks:** Two times per week—Tuesday and Thursday

These workouts build foundational endurance and strength. Stick to the recommended workout time. If you want a greater challenge, experiment with heavier weight, faster speed, or incline to increase intensity, or add strength movements using your rucksack before, during, or after the ruck.

**Long ruck:** One day per week—Saturday

A longer session helps you prepare for the endurance needed to complete a 5K and get mileage under your feet. Maintain a steady pace and good form throughout. Using a lighter ruck weight can help prevent unnecessary strain. Change it up with new trails or scenery to keep it fresh and inspiring.

**Strength training:** Optional, one or two times per week—Monday and/or Friday

Focus on full-body compound exercises such as squats, lunges, planks, and rows. These sessions help build muscle and improve your ability to carry weight over time. If you're new to exercise, wait until Week 3 or 4 to add strength training to the mix.

**Mobility work:** Optional, one or two times per week—Wednesday and/or Sunday

Stretching, yoga, or foam rolling help improve flexibility and reduce muscle aches, aiding recovery. You can add mobility work to any day or after any ruck. Even a five-minute stretch feels great for sore muscles.

**Rest days:** Rest drives recovery and allows your body time to adapt to new stressors. The program includes a generous number of optional rest days. If you're a beginner, take them. Tune in to your body and remember that rest is productive. If, at any point, the strain of walking with weight feels like too much, drop the pack and just go for a walk. Walking gets the blood flowing, accrues steps, and keeps you on pace with the training plan. Some days will feel easier than others. Adapt, but don't quit.

# 10K TRAINING PROGRAM

Like the 5K program, this training regimen takes place over eight weeks but with longer distances, faster progression, and an end goal of 10K (6.2 miles). Consider this plan if you're new to rucking but not new to regular exercise. You should have an aerobic base and the ability to tolerate the workload to avoid setbacks, such as overuse injuries.

## *Overview*

| Week | Rucks per Week | Duration | Distance | Weight | Focus |
|------|------|----------|----------|--------|-------|
| 1 | 2 or 3 | 30–45 minutes | 1–2 miles | 10–20 pounds | posture, walking under load |
| 2 | 3 | 45 minutes | 2 miles | 10–20 pounds | increased pace and distance |
| 3 | 3 | 45 minutes–1 hour | 2–3 miles | 10–25 pounds | slight hills or varied terrain for 1 ruck |
| 4 | 3 | 1 hour | 3 miles | 15–30 pounds | 15–20 minutes per mile for 1 ruck |
| 5 | 3 | 1–1¼ hours | 3–4 miles | 15–30 pounds | plus 10–15 minutes strength exercises after 1 short ruck |
| 6 | 3 or 4 | 1¼–1½ hours | 4–5 miles | 15–30 pounds | nutrition strategies to fuel performance (Chapter 5) |
| 7 | 3 or 4 | 1½–2 hours | 5–6 miles | 20–40 pounds | maintaining pace for longer distances, nutrition, and hydration |
| 8 | 2 or 3 | 2 hours | 6 miles | 20–40 pounds | tapering to complete the 10K |

## Sample Workout Calendar

Because this plan calls for longer rucks and higher intensity, take the rest days. Feel free to adjust the days to fit your weekly routine but aim to maintain the structure of rucking, rest, and optional cross-training to optimize recovery and progress.

| Day | Weeks 1–4 | Weeks 5–6 | Weeks 7–8 |
|---|---|---|---|
| Monday | strength training or rest | strength training or rest | strength training or rest |
| Tuesday | regular ruck 30 minutes–1 hour | regular ruck 1–1½ hours | regular ruck, 1½–2 hours |
| Wednesday | mobility work or rest | mobility work or rest | mobility work or rest |
| Thursday | regular ruck, 30 minutes–1 hour | regular ruck, 40 minutes–1 hour | lightweight ruck, 1–2 hours |
| Friday | strength training or rest | strength training or rest | strength training or rest |
| Saturday | long ruck, 1–3 miles | long ruck, 3–5 miles | long ruck, 5–6.2 miles |
| Sunday | mobility work or rest | mobility work or rest | mobility work or rest |

## Components

**Regular rucks:** Two times per week—Tuesday and Thursday

These workouts build foundational endurance and strength. Stick to the recommended workout time. If you want a greater challenge, experiment with heavier weight, faster speed, or incline to increase intensity, or add strength movements using your rucksack before, during, or after the ruck.

**Long ruck:** One day per week—Saturday

As the cornerstone of the plan, this ruck progressively builds endurance to complete the 10K. Maintain a steady pace and good form throughout. Using a lighter ruck weight can help prevent unnecessary strain. Change it up with new trails or scenery to keep it fresh and inspiring.

**Strength training:** Optional, one or two times per week—Monday and/or Friday

Focus on full-body compound exercises such as squats, lunges, presses, and rows. For a greater challenge, incorporate explosive power movements, including box jumps, kettlebell swings, or other plyometric movements between compound lifts to increase power and speed. Limit power movements to one strength session per week.

**Mobility work:** Optional, one or two times per week—Wednesday and/or Sunday

Stretching, yoga, or foam rolling help improve flexibility and reduce muscle aches, aiding recovery. You can add mobility work to any day or after any ruck to ease sore muscles.

**Rest days:** At least one day per week

Include a minimum of one full rest day in Weeks 5 to 8 when longer, more intense rucks become more frequent. Walking without weight still gets the blood flowing and counts as active recovery. Listen to your body and remember that rest builds resilience.

# HALF-MARATHON OR 25K TRAINING PROGRAM

Rucking a half-marathon (13.1 miles, 21K) or a 25K (15.5 miles) requires substantial physical and mental preparation. Choose this plan if you already have a solid fitness base and experience with rucking or endurance activities.

Unlike the first two plans, this one gives no weight recommendations. The higher demands of the program require using knowledge of your own body to find a ruck weight and training intensities that work for you. These will likely vary from session to session, based on distance and duration. For example, short rucks may be heavier while long rucks may be lighter. This training plan goes hard on mileage, so don't ruck heavy every single time.

This program requires more than double the distance, time, and dedication of the 10K option, so complete the 10K plan before taking on this challenge. More time on your feet means more opportunity to overtrain, so pay attention to your body for signs of chronic fatigue, irritability, trouble sleeping, and other considerations discussed in Chapter 2. Before you begin, keep these key points in mind:

**Consistency:** Training for a half-marathon or 25K requires lots of time under load and a disciplined approach to weekly rucking, strength training, and recovery. Plan wisely but remain flexible. Life happens. If you miss a day, don't let it derail the whole program. Keep moving and don't worry about executing the plan to a T.

**Fuel and hydration:** Paying attention to nutrition and hydration help you avoid "bonking" (or "hitting the wall," which is sudden fatigue from underfueling) and cutting your sessions short. You might use supplements to power through long workouts. More about fueling for long rucks in Chapter 5.

**Mental toughness:** Not every workout will feel easy or enjoyable, and the distance will test your resilience. A marathoner client of mine embraces the rule of thirds for her training: a third of sessions will suck, a third will be OK, and a third will feel great. Setting realistic expectations, like the rule of thirds, helps avoid discouragement later in the program. It's not supposed to be easy.

**Tapering:** If you signed up for an event, taper your training in Weeks 11 and 12. Gradually reducing mileage and intensity allows your body time to recover so you feel refreshed and ready to perform on race day.

## Overview

| Week | Rucks per Week | Long Ruck | Other Rucks | Focus |
|------|------|------|------|------|
| 1 | 2 or 3 | 4 miles | 2–3 miles | form and consistency |
| 2 | 3 | 5 miles | 2–3 miles | increase pace for shorter rucks |
| 3 | 3 | 6 miles | 3 miles | add 15–20 minutes strength training after 1 short ruck |
| 4 | 3 | 7 miles | 3–4 miles | hills or intervals for 1 short ruck |
| 5 | 3 | 8 miles | 3–4 miles | practice pacing, nutrition, and hydration for long ruck (Chapter 5) |
| 6 | 3 | 9 miles | 4 miles | simulate racecourse terrain for the long ruck |
| 7 | 3 | 10 miles | 4–5 miles | 15–20 minutes per mile for the long ruck |
| 8 | 3 | 11 miles | 4–5 miles | nutrition strategy for the long ruck |
| 9 | 3 | 12 miles | 4–6 miles | breathing, cadence, and other rhythms |
| 10 | 3 | 13–14 miles | 5–6 miles | long ruck as full-race simulation |
| 11 | 3 | 10 miles | 4–5 miles | tapering training volume while maintaining consistency |
| 12 | 2 or 3 | 15.5 miles | 2–5 miles | further tapering, rest, and mobility work for optimal performance on race day |

## Sample Workout Calendar

Because this plan calls for lots of lengthy rucks, focus on upper body exercises and compound lower body movements on strength days to keep your legs fresh for long-ruck days.

| Day | Weeks 1–4 | Weeks 5–8 | Weeks 9–11 | Week 12 |
|---|---|---|---|---|
| Monday | strength training or mobility work | strength training or mobility work | strength training or mobility work | regular ruck, 2–5 miles |
| Tuesday | regular ruck, 2–4 miles | regular ruck, 3–5 miles | regular ruck, 4–6 miles | mobility work or rest |
| Wednesday | strength training | strength training | strength training | regular ruck, 2–5 miles |
| Thursday | regular ruck, 3–4 miles | regular ruck, 4–5 miles | regular ruck, 5–6 miles | mobility work or rest |
| Friday | mobility work or rest | mobility work or rest | mobility work or rest | mobility work or rest |
| Saturday | long ruck, 4–7 miles | long ruck, 8–11 miles | long ruck, 12–15.5 miles | long ruck, 13.1–15.5 miles |
| Sunday | mobility work or rest | mobility work or rest | mobility work or rest | mobility work or rest |

## Components

**Regular rucks:** Two times per week—Tuesday and Thursday

These workouts build foundational endurance and strength. Stick to the recommended workout time. If you want a greater challenge, experiment with heavier weight, faster speed, or incline to increase intensity. You could also add strength movements using your rucksack before, during, or after the ruck.

**Long ruck:** One day per week—Saturday

As the cornerstone of the plan, this ruck progressively builds endurance to complete the 25K or half-marathon distance. Maintain a steady pace and good form throughout. Using a lighter ruck weight can help prevent unnecessary strain. Change it up with new trails or scenery to keep it fresh and inspiring. Test hydration and nutrition strategies, so you have a solid fueling plan on race day.

**Strength training:** One or two times per week—Monday and/or Wednesday

Focus on full-body and upper body movements. If you need to rearrange training days, don't do a heavy strength day and long-ruck day back-to-back.

**Mobility work:** Up to three times per week—Monday, Friday, and/or Sunday

This training counts as active recovery. Stretching, yoga, or foam rolling help improve flexibility and reduce muscle aches, aiding recovery.

**Rest days:** One or two days per week

Include a minimum of one full rest day, especially in Weeks 7 to 12, when longer, more intense rucks hit double-digit mileage. Listen to your body and remember that rest is productive.

## *Tapering for Race Day*

If you're training for an official half-marathon or 25K ruck event, tapering will ensure proper rest so you're ready to perform at your peak on race day. Tapering is an intentional reduction in training volume during the final week or two before your event. Here's how to taper effectively:

**Reduce mileage.** Gradually decrease the duration and distance of your rucks during the last one or two weeks of the program. Rucking *and* strength sessions should run shorter and lighter.

**Maintain frequency.** Continue rucking two or three times per week but keep the effort light to stay loose and prevent stiffness.

**Focus on recovery.** Prioritize rest and mobility work during the taper period to give your body time to recuperate. Come race day, you won't regret the extra downtime.

**Practice good nutrition.** Well before race day, lock in your fuel and hydration strategies. The day of the event is not the time to experiment with new pre-workout meals or supplements. See Chapter 5 for specific nutrition guidelines.

## STRENGTH TRAINING

To maximize your fitness potential, strength training must be a part of the equation, and it doesn't have to be complicated. Building a durable body doesn't require hours in the gym or fancy equipment. All you need is your ruck.

A rucksack can easily substitute for traditional weight training equipment, including barbells or dumbbells. Its cost-effectiveness and portability make it an excellent option for the gym, home workouts, outdoor training, and even travel. By adjusting the ruck weight, you can tailor the resistance to your fitness level and gradually build muscle and strength.

Unlike isolated movements or machines, rucksack exercises mimic real-world activities, such as climbing stairs or lifting objects, making your gains more applicable to everyday life. Squats or step-ups with a ruck—rather than holding the weight on your shoulders or in your hands—change your center of gravity and provide a different challenge for your body. While there's no right way to organize your routine, here is one of my favorite and most efficient ways to plan your training.

## The Push-Pull-Leg (PPL) Split

The world of strength training features many "splits"—meaning how you arrange your strength sessions throughout the week—such as upper-and-lower body days, full-body routines, and body-part-specific workouts. The push-pull-leg (PPL) split stands out for its balance and efficiency.

Unlike muscle-specific splits, PPL routines target larger movement patterns and muscle groups, which leads to better overall muscle development and strength gains. You train smarter and more strategically by grouping workouts into the following segments:

**Push day:** These movements push weight away from your body. Muscles involved include the chest, shoulders, and triceps.

**Pull day:** These movements pull weight toward your body. Muscles involved include the back and biceps.

**Leg day:** These movements focus on lower body strength. Muscles involved include the quads, hamstrings, glutes, and calves.

Compound movements—such as squats, deadlifts, and push-ups—serve as cornerstone exercises in PPL routines. Compound movements engage multiple muscle groups simultaneously, improving coordination and saving time compared to training each body part individually. For example, a squat targets the quads while activating the hamstrings, glutes, lower back, and core. In contrast, a leg extension machine focuses solely on quads, offering less overall functional benefit. Targeting individual muscles helps bodybuilders accentuate specific areas of the body, but compound movements complement how we function in the real world. Compound movements also burn more calories and build strength faster than isolation exercises, making them incredibly efficient. They create maximum gains in minimal time.

A PPL regimen also makes the most of recovery time, allowing you to train as frequently as you'd like. For example, the muscles in a push day—chest, shoulders, and triceps—are recovering while you focus on your next workout, either a pull day or leg day. This strategic balance reduces the risk of overtraining and promotes long-term consistency while allowing you to seamlessly integrate your strength routine into your weekly routine.

Following a PPL split doesn't have to entail three training days per week, either. Use the framework to increase or decrease training days to accommodate what works for you. For example, if you want to condense weight training into two days, as many of the *Ruck Fit* training plans do, add squats to push day and deadlifts to pull day to create a full-body workout that targets all major muscle groups over the course of a week. Alternatively, you might opt for shorter, more frequent sessions, such as three to five strength workouts per week, rotating through the movement patterns. You can also stack a few strength exercises before or after your rucks.

To formulate a training regimen that works for you, mix and

match exercises from the following menu, which includes core movements to complement strength-training sessions and aid trunk stability.

| Push | Pull | Legs | Core |
|---|---|---|---|
| bench press | pull-ups | squats | plank |
| push-ups | rows | deadlifts | side plank |
| overhead press | lat pulldown | lunges | Russian twists |
| chest press | deadlifts | step-ups | bicycle crunches |
| chest flys | bicep curls | calf raises | leg raises |
| dips | lateral raise | sled push | mountain climbers |

**Push, pull, or leg workout:** Choose two or three movements from the specific category. Add one or two core exercises, if desired.

**Full-body workout:** Mix and match one or two leg and core exercises each, with two or three push or pull movements.

Perform two to four sets of 6 to 12 reps of each exercise. By the end of the set (near the top-end of the rep range), you should feel like you could muster out just one or two more reps with good form, for optimal results. Apply progressive overload by gradually increasing weight or reps each week.

Don't stress about designing the perfect strength-training plan. What matters is that you're moving weight safely and effectively. To bring it all together, here's how to incorporate a rucksack into a PPL routine.

## PUSH DAY

**Push-ups with rucksack:** Wear your ruck while performing push-ups (page 98).

**Overhead presses with rucksack:** Hold the ruck by its ends and press it overhead (page 100).

**Dips with rucksack:** Wear your rucksack and perform dips using parallel bars or any sturdy, stable surface (page 102).

## PULL DAY

**Rucksack rows:** Leaning toward the floor, hold the ruck by its ends and pull it toward your midsection (page 104).

**Upright rows with rucksack:** Grip the straps of the rucksack and, with the ruck hanging in front of you, pull up until your arms are parallel to the ground (page 106).

**Bicep curls with rucksack:** Use a rucksack as a makeshift weight for curls by gripping the ends of the pack or using the handles (page 108).

**Pull-ups:** If you have a pull-up bar, wear your ruck while performing pull-ups or chin-ups.

## LEG DAY

**Squats with rucksack:** Wear your ruck and squat. For a greater challenge, hold additional weight, such as sandbags, weight plates, or any heavy object (page 110).

**Lunges with rucksack:** Wear your rucksack while performing stationary or walking lunges. Modify the movement to the back and sides or rotate among all three (page 114).

**Deadlifts with rucksack:** Use a rucksack to mimic the motion of a traditional deadlift, focusing on keeping your spine neutral and engaging your hamstrings and glutes (page 118).

**Step-ups with rucksack:** Wear a ruck while you step onto a platform, plyometric box, or staircase (page 121).

# STRENGTH EXERCISES

This section showcases step-by-step instructions for some of my favorite exercises using a ruck to build muscle, improve functional strength, and create a balanced, capable body.

## PUSH-UPS WITH RUCKSACK

This exercise strengthens the chest, shoulders, triceps, and core. With proper form and thoughtful progressions, a push-up can be modified to suit any fitness level to develop upper body strength.

**Starting position:** Lying face down, place your hands under your shoulders, fingers pointing forward. Press your body away from the ground with legs extended in a high plank position. Engage your core and tuck your pelvis, keeping your body straight from head to heels.

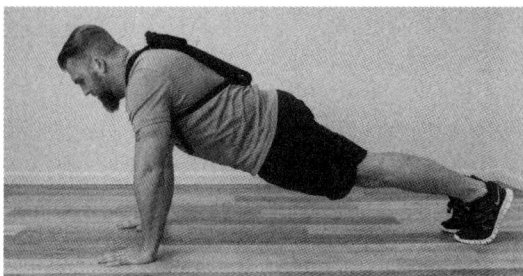

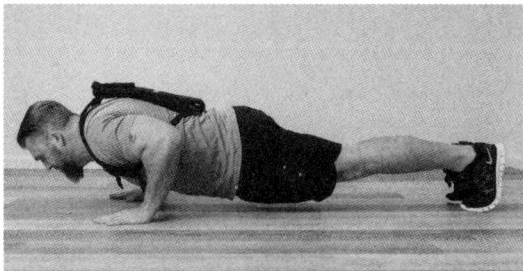

**Movement:** Inhale as you lower your chest to the ground by bending at the elbows, keeping them tucked close to your torso. Stop when your chest is just above the ground or your elbows form a 90-degree angle. Exhale as you push through your palms to return to the starting position, maintaining straight and stable alignment throughout the movement.

**Variations:** *Diamond/close-grip/triceps push-up:* For the starting position, bring your hands together so your thumbs and index fingers form a diamond shape. Keep your elbows close to your ribs ensuring they don't flare out. This hand placement shifts emphasis from the chest to the triceps.

*Wide-grip push-up:* Place your hands wider than shoulder-width apart to increase the stretch and activation of the chest muscles.

**Make it easier:**
- Keep your knees on the ground for knee push-ups.
- Perform incline push-ups by placing your hands on a sturdy, elevated surface such as a bench, step, or wall.
- Remove the ruck for bodyweight push-ups.
- Do negative push-ups by slowly lowering yourself to the ground before returning to the starting position.

**Make it harder:**
- Add more weight to your rucksack while maintaining proper form.
- Do decline push-ups with your feet elevated on a bench or step.
- Pause at the bottom of the movement for two or three seconds to increase time under tension.
- Perform plyometric push-ups by explosively pushing off the ground, allowing your hands to leave the floor briefly.

## OVERHEAD PRESSES WITH RUCKSACK

Pressing a ruck overhead strengthens the deltoids, trapezius, triceps, and upper chest while working on balance and coordination. This functional exercise can help with everyday tasks, such as changing lightbulbs or loading luggage into an overhead compartment.

**Starting position:** Hold the rucksack securely by its ends. Stand with your feet shoulder-width apart, knees slightly bent, core engaged. Keep the ruck close to your chest, with your elbows bent and ruck parallel to the ground.

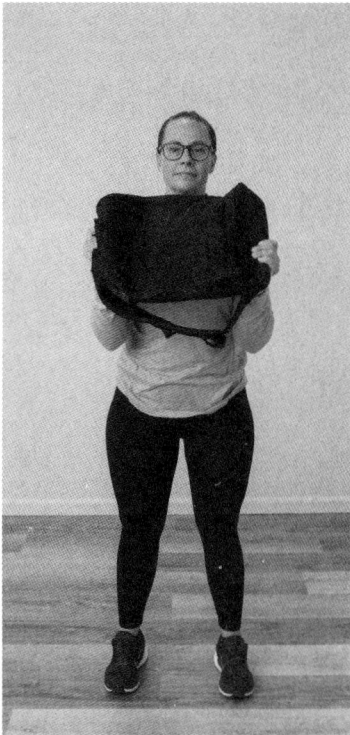

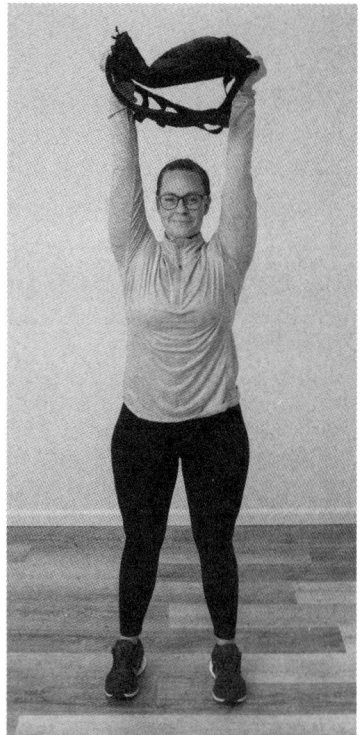

**Movement:** Brace your core, keeping your spine neutral. Press the ruck overhead, extending your arms fully without locking your elbows. Slowly lower the ruck back to chest level and repeat.

**Make it easier:**

- Reduce the ruck weight.
- Sit on a bench or chair to minimize core and lower body involvement.
- Add a slight push-press by bending your knees and using a small leg drive to move the weight overhead.

**Make it harder:**

- Add weight to your ruck.
- Incorporate a squat before pressing the ruck overhead to complete a "thruster."

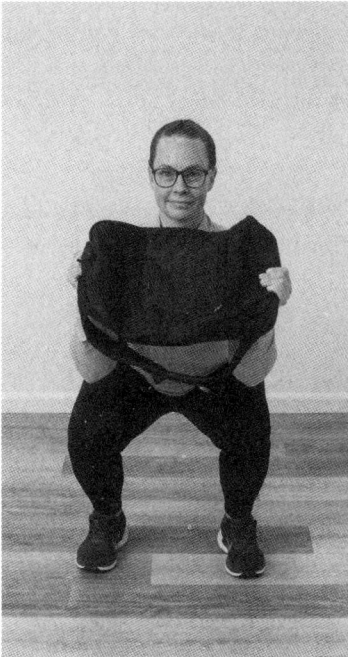

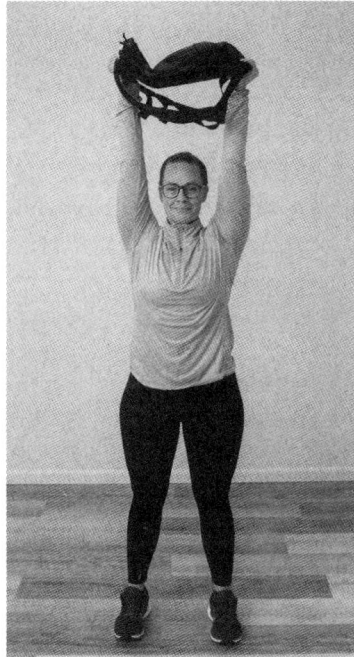

## DIPS WITH RUCKSACK

As a functional exercise, dips help with pushing yourself up off the floor or from a seated position. A rucksack increases resistance, making the movement more challenging and effective for building muscle and shoulder stability.

**Starting position:** Position yourself on a sturdy surface such as a bench or parallel bars. On parallel bars, grip the bars with your arms fully extended at your sides, supporting your body in a vertical position. On a bench, place your palms behind you, fingers facing forward. In either variation, keep your chest upright, shoulders back, and core engaged.

**Movement:** Bend your elbows, keeping them close to your sides, as you lower your body. Dip until your upper arms are nearly parallel to the ground, depending on your shoulder mobility. Pause briefly, then press through your palms to straighten your arms and return to the starting position.

**Make it easier:**
- Perform without a ruck.
- Use an assisted dip machine or resistance bands looped under your knees (if using parallel bars) to reduce the load on your arms.
- Lower yourself only partway.

**Make it harder:**
- Add more weight to your ruck.
- Place your feet on an elevated surface, such as a bench or step, to challenge your core and balance.
- Use a weighted belt or hold a dumbbell between your legs.

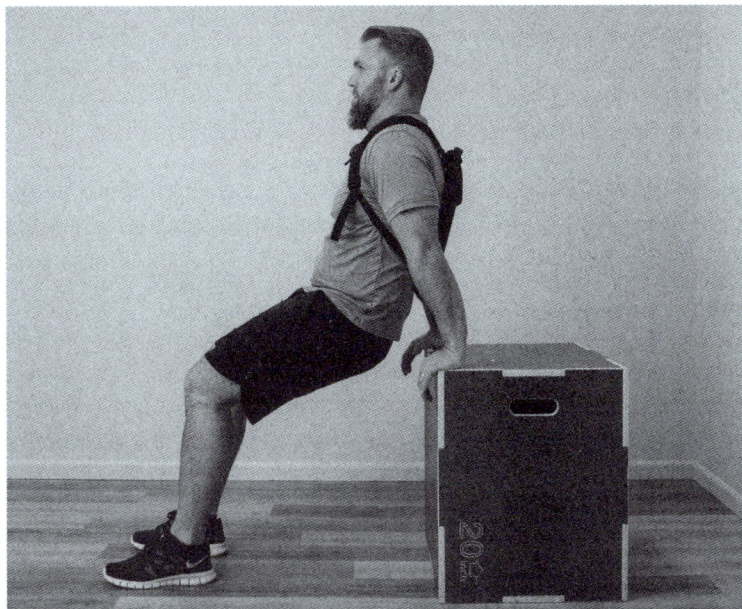

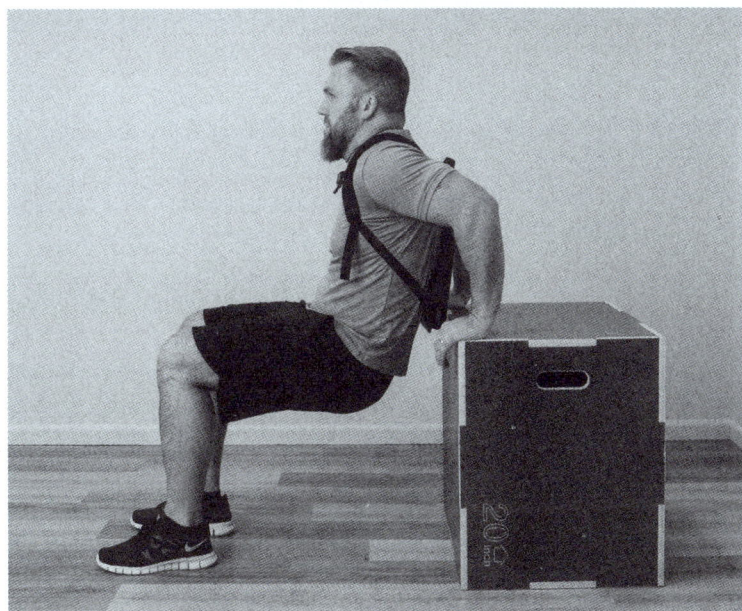

## RUCKSACK ROWS

This movement targets pulling muscles, helping to improve posture, enhance grip strength, and create a balanced upper body.

**Starting position:** Stand with your feet shoulder-width apart and your torso at a 45-degree angle to the ground. Keep your back straight and core engaged. With your arms hanging below your shoulders, grip your ruck securely by the ends or by the top and bottom handles.

**Movement:** Pull the ruck toward your torso, drawing your elbows back while keeping them close to your body. At the top of the

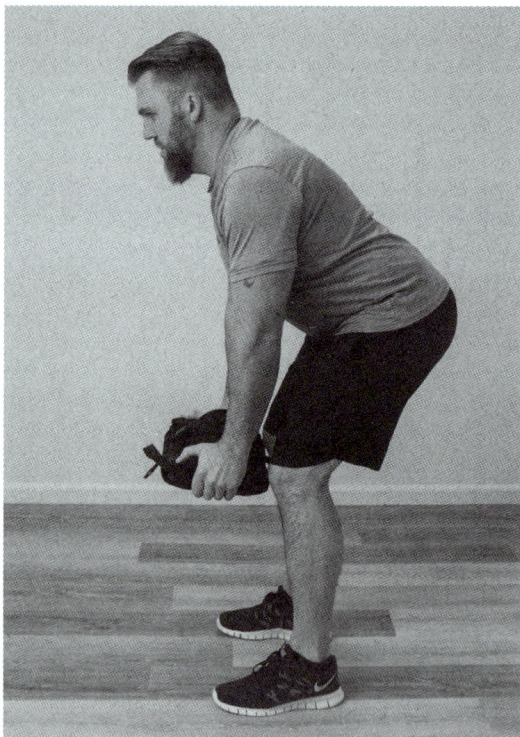

movement, squeeze your shoulder blades together before lowering the ruck back to the starting position, maintaining control throughout.

**Make it easier:**
- Reduce the weight of your ruck.

**Make it harder:**
- Increase the weight of your ruck.
- After each row, add a deadlift.
- Hold the ruck by the handle with one hand instead of two, performing the movement unilaterally to challenge your balance and core stability.

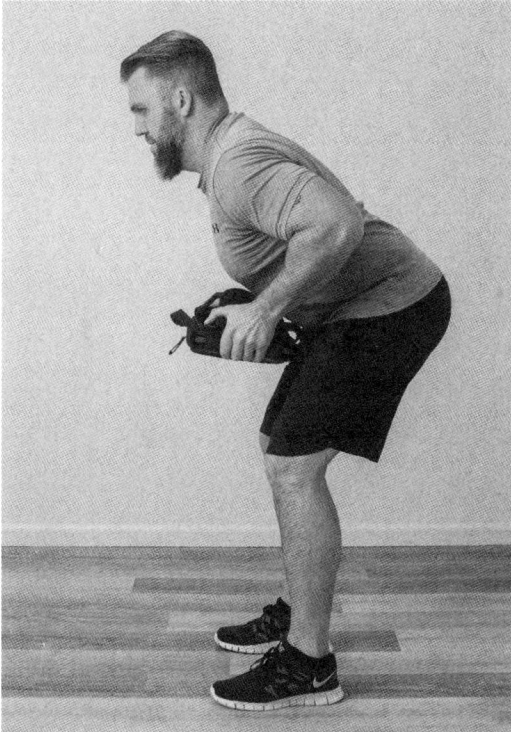

## UPRIGHT ROWS WITH RUCKSACK

This movement helps improve posture, shoulder strength, and overall upper body symmetry. When you build bigger traps, you create a natural cushion for your ruck to rest on.

**Starting position:** Stand with your feet shoulder-width apart, knees slightly bent. Using both hands, hold the rucksack by its top handle or by the straps, palms facing in. With arms fully extended, let the ruck hang in front of you.

**Movement:** Pull the rucksack up toward your chest by drawing your elbows upward and outward. Pull with your elbows, rather than your hands, to engage the correct muscles. Keep the ruck

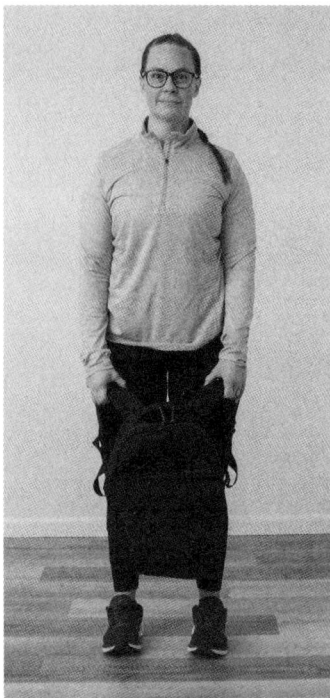

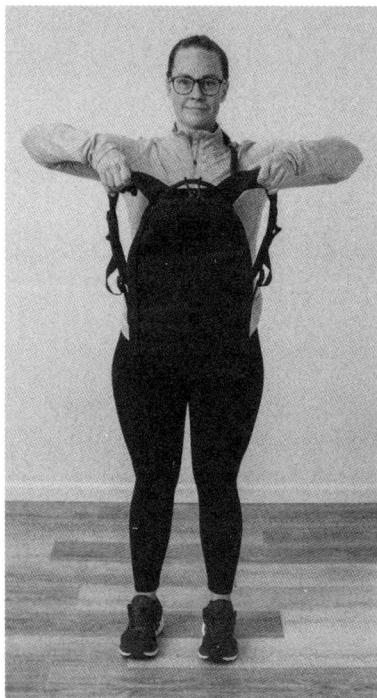

close to your body throughout the movement. Stop when your elbows reach shoulder height or are just parallel to the ground. Slowly lower the ruck back to the starting position.

**Make it easier:**
- Reduce the ruck weight.
- Pull the ruck only partway up.

**Make it harder:**
- Increase the ruck weight.
- Incorporate a deadlift before pulling the ruck into position to complete a "high-pull" (below).

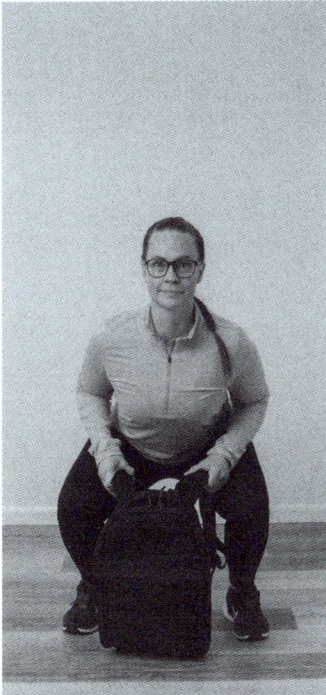

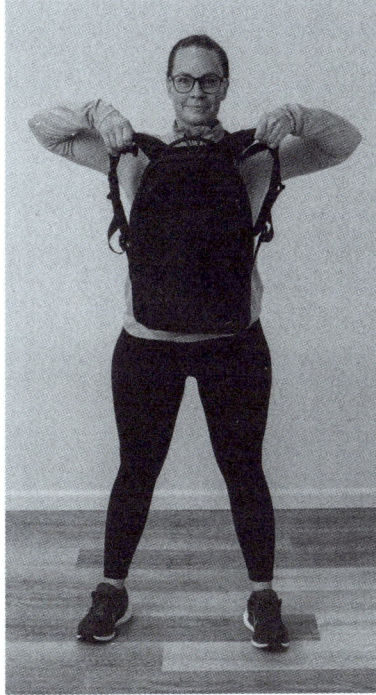

## BICEP CURLS WITH RUCKSACK

A rucksack makes this simple yet effective exercise for building arm strength, improving grip, and toning the biceps a versatile option for all fitness levels. Various grips adapt the movement to target different muscles of the arm.

**Starting position:** Stand upright with your feet shoulder-width apart. Hold the rucksack by its ends with palms facing in. Let your arms hang naturally in front of you with a slight bend in your elbows.

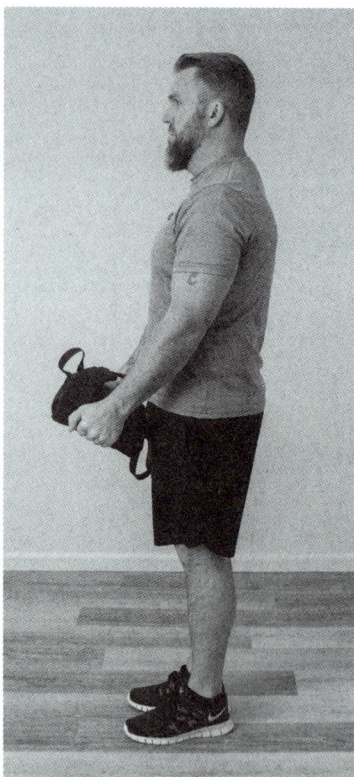

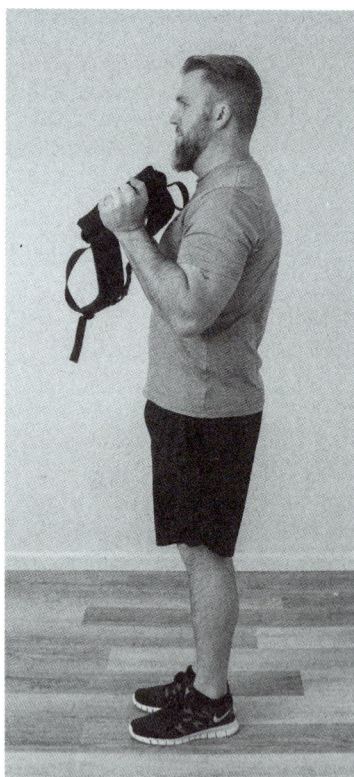

**Movement:** Bend your elbows and curl the ruck to your chest, keeping your upper arms and elbows tucked close to your sides. Don't swing the ruck. Use controlled movements and avoid using momentum from your hips or shoulders. Squeeze your biceps at the top of the movement before slowly lowering to the starting position.

**Make it easier:**

- Reduce the ruck weight.
- Limit the range of motion by curling the ruck only halfway up or down.
- Sit on a bench or chair to focus your attention on just your arms and biceps.

**Make it harder:**

- Add weight to your ruck.
- Hold the ruck with one hand, by its top handle, and curl it unilaterally.
- Pause halfway through the curl and hold for two or three seconds before completing the movement.
- After curling the ruck to chest level, push the weight up into an overhead press and turn the movement into a compound exercise.

## SQUATS WITH RUCKSACK

This powerful exercise builds lower body strength, improves trunk stability, and enhances overall endurance—all while mimicking functional movements of daily life, such as squatting to pick something off the floor or standing from a seated position. Movement patterns such as this help maintain independence as you age.

**Starting position:** Stand with your feet shoulder-width apart or slightly wider, depending on your natural stance. Keep your chest upright and shoulders pulled down and back. Imagine tucking your shoulder blades into your back pockets. Keep your gaze forward and brace your core, as if you're preparing to absorb a light punch to your stomach, keeping your spine neutral and protecting your lower back.

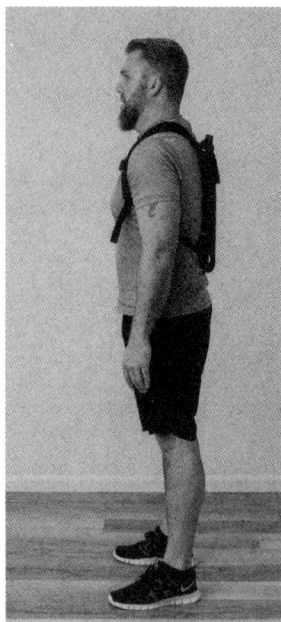

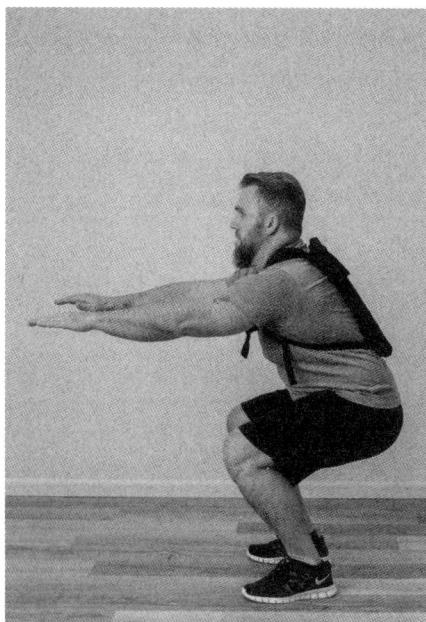

**Movement:** Bend at your hips, pushing your butt back as if you were sitting into a chair. As you lower your body, keep your chest upright and extend your arms forward to create counterbalance for the ruck weight. Keep your knees in line with your toes and don't let them collapse inward. Imagine pressing your knees outward for added stability. Lower your hips until your thighs run parallel to the ground or as far as your mobility allows without rounding your lower back. Pause at the bottom of the movement, then press firmly through your heels and return to the starting position, squeezing your glutes at the top for full hip extension. Keep the motion slow and controlled throughout.

**Variations:** *Front squat:* This modification targets the front thighs, or quads. Wear your ruck backward—on your chest rather than your back—or hold it firmly in front of you with your elbows bent and weight close to your chest. Keep your spine neutral throughout the movement.

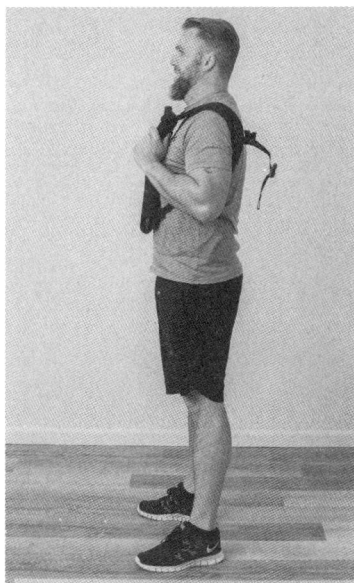

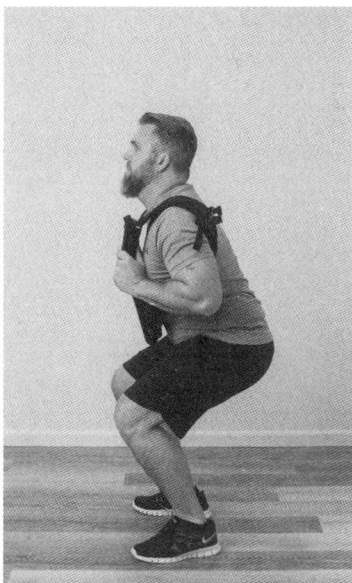

*Wide stance:* A wider stance increases activation of the inner thigh muscles and glutes, making it an excellent option for improving hip mobility. Start with your feet wider than shoulder-width apart. Point your toes outward at a 30- to 45-degree angle, depending on your hip mobility. As you sumo-squat down, engage your glutes to prevent your knees from caving in.

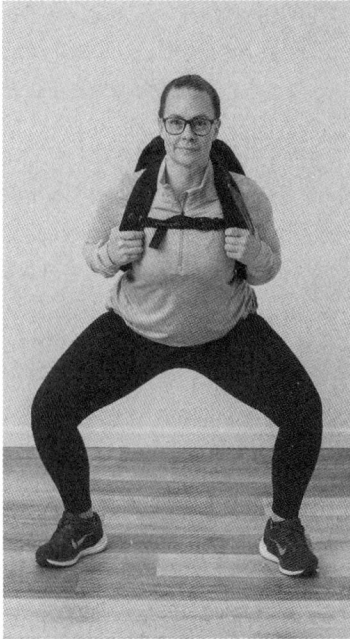

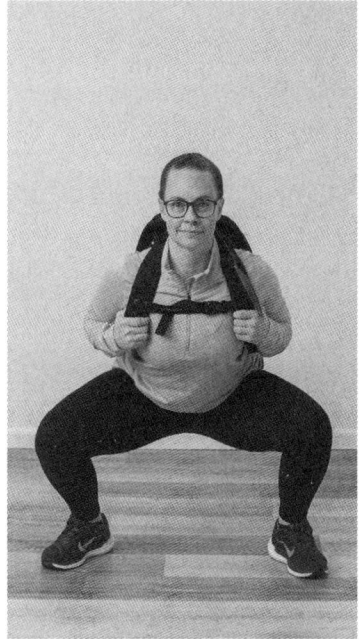

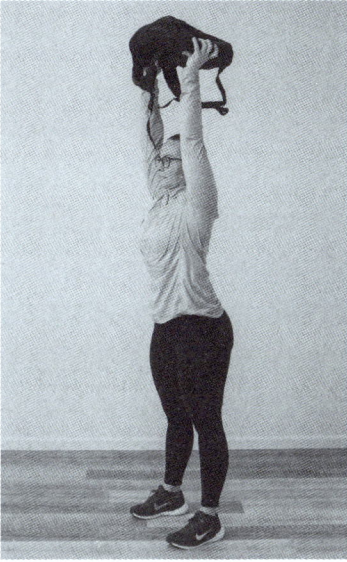

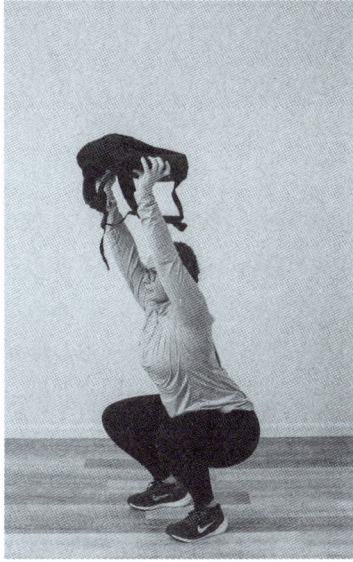

*Overhead squat:* Challenge your balance and core strength by holding the weight overhead for a full-body exercise. Grab your ruck by its ends and extend it above your head, locking your elbows at the top. Brace your core to protect your spine as you lower into a squat position.

*Narrow stance:* This version shifts emphasis to the quads. Start with your feet narrower than shoulder-width apart. Point your toes forward with enough room between your feet to place a fist.

**Make it easier:**
- Omit the ruck and use only your body weight.
- For extra support, squat into a chair or try holding on to a railing.

**Make it harder:**
- Increase the ruck weight or hold on to dumbbells, kettlebells, or sandbags while maintaining good form.
- Add pulses to the bottom of the movement for extra burn.

## LUNGES WITH RUCKSACK

This dynamic exercise challenges your lower body strength and stability. Lunges can also help correct muscle imbalances between the left and right legs.

**Starting position:** Stand upright with your feet hip-width apart and engage your core for stability.

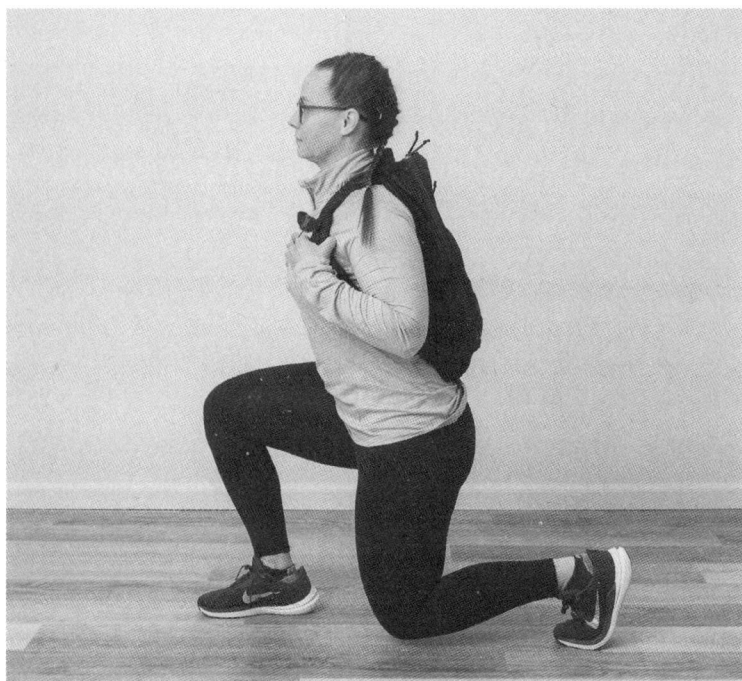

**Movement:** Step one foot forward into a lunge, lowering your hips until your back knee is just above the ground or as low as your mobility allows. Keep your chest upright and your front knee aligned over your front foot. Push through your front heel to return to the starting position and repeat on the opposite leg.

**Variations:** *Reverse lunge:* Reverse lunges are easier on the knees and offer a great way to strengthen the glutes and hamstrings. Start with your feet hip-width apart. Instead of stepping forward, step one foot backward into a lunge while lowering your back knee toward the ground.

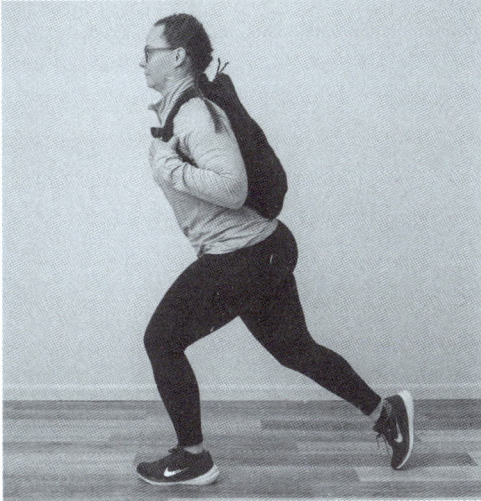

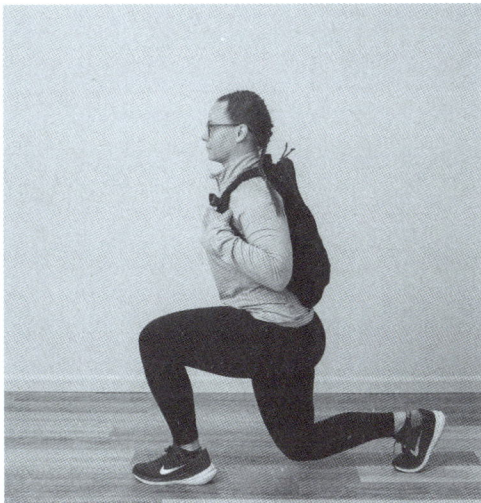

*Side lunge:* Lateral lunges improve hip mobility and strengthen muscles used in side-to-side motions, a plane of movement that's often overlooked in traditional workouts. Start with your feet wider than shoulder-width apart. Shift your weight to one side, bending the knee while keeping the other leg straight. Push your hips back as you lower into the lunge, ensuring your bent knee tracks over your toes. Keep your chest upright, core engaged, and bring your arms in front of you as a counterbalance.

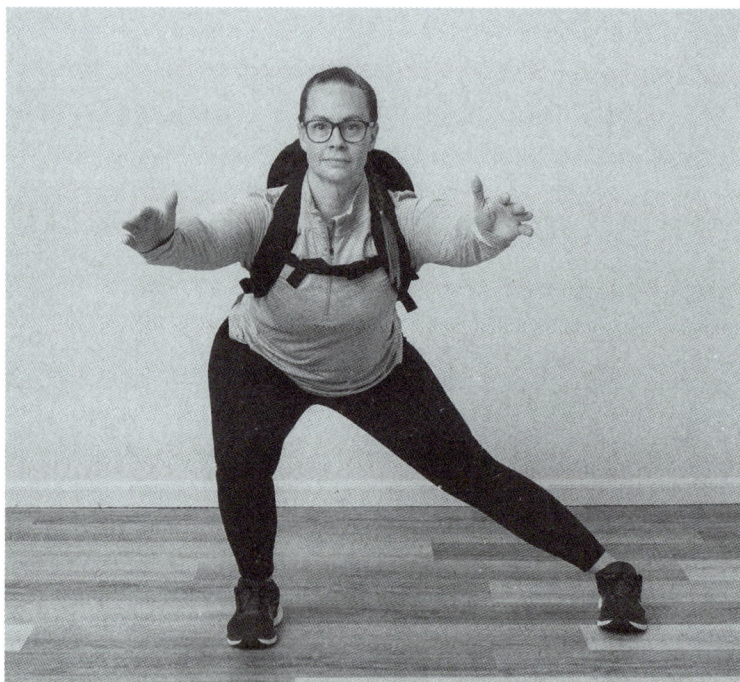

## Make it easier:

- Use only your body weight.
- Hold on to a sturdy object such as a chair, wall, or rail for added stability.

## Make it harder:

- Add weight to your ruck or hold on to dumbbells, kettlebells, or sandbags while maintaining good form.
- Pick up the tempo and, instead of returning to the starting position, step forward with the other leg to perform continuous walking lunges.
- Pause or pulse at the bottom of the lunge for two or three seconds to increase time under tension.
- Combine forward, lateral, and reverse lunges to challenge your muscles in all planes of motion. For example, do a forward lunge followed by a lateral and rear lunge on your right leg before transitioning through the same sequence on your left leg.

## DEADLIFTS WITH RUCKSACK

This foundational exercise strengthens the posterior chain—glutes, hamstrings, and lower back—while engaging the core and upper body. Adding a ruck makes it a functional movement, simulating real-world activities such as picking up heavy objects. This is my favorite of the leg movements.

**Starting position:** Place your ruck on the ground in front of you, between your feet. Stand with your feet wider than hip-width apart with your toes pointing forward.

**Movement:** With a flat back, push your hips back and down, as if you were sitting back into a chair, and grip the ends of the ruck with both hands. Keep your arms straight and core engaged as you

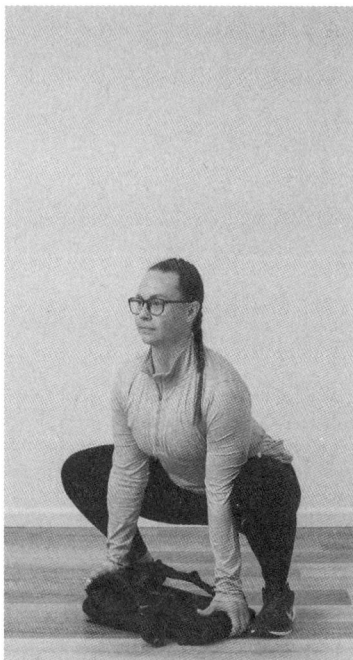

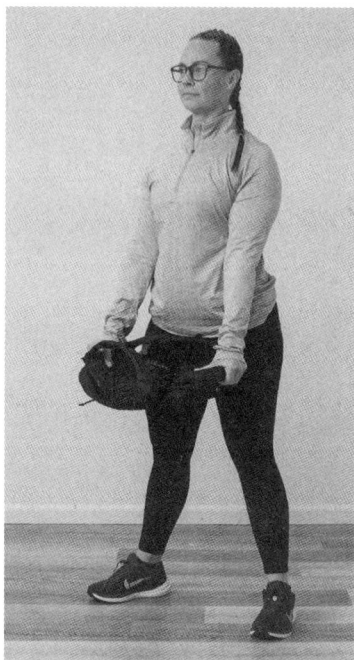

lift the ruck off the ground. Drive through your heels, pressing your hips forward and squeezing your butt at the top of the movement. Lower the ruck back to the ground by hinging at your hips and bending your knees, keeping the ruck close to your body. If it helps, think *dead-pull* and imagine pushing the floor away with your feet to cue the correct muscles.

**Variations:** *Romanian/stiff-leg deadlift:* Begin by standing upright, with the ruck in your hands. Keep your feet about hip-width apart and your knees slightly bent. Push your hips back as if closing a door with your glutes, maintaining a neutral spine and keeping your chest proud. Lower the weight without touching the ground. Imagine shaving your shins with your ruck to keep the weight close to the midline.

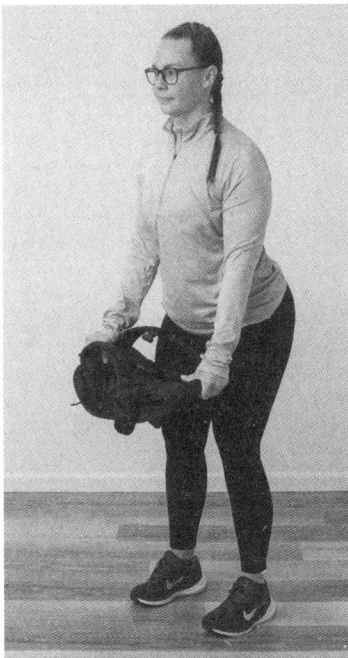

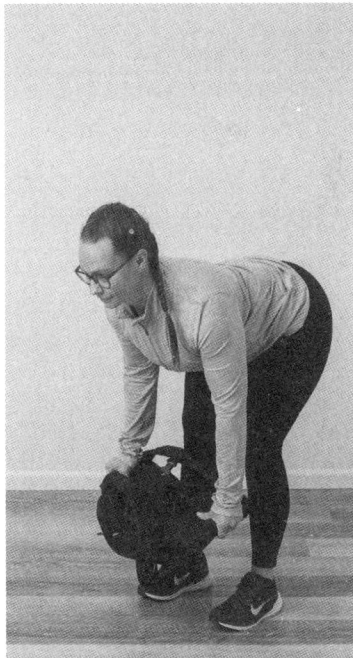

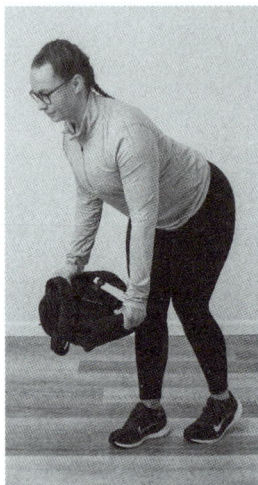

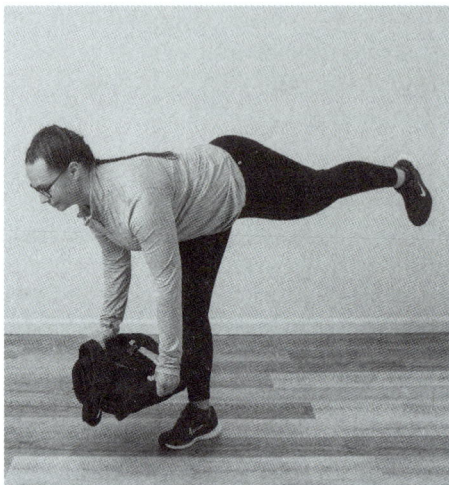

*Single-leg deadlift:* Shift your weight to one leg. As you bend down, extend the opposite leg behind you as a counterbalance.

**Make it easier:**
- Start with the ruck on a raised platform (step or box) to reduce the range of motion.
- Lower the ruck partway instead of all the way to the ground.

**Make it harder:**
- Add extra weight to your ruck.
- Add a high-pull to the movement by picking up your ruck from the top handle and incorporating an upright row.

## STEP-UPS WITH RUCKSACK

This movement emulates climbing stairs or hiking steep trails, making it one of the most functional and practical lower body exercises you can do. Adding a rucksack elevates the challenge by loading your body and engaging your core, transforming this simple motion into a scalable movement suitable for all fitness levels.

**Starting position:** Stand in front of a sturdy surface, such as a box, bench, or step that's knee-height or lower. When your foot is on the surface, your knee should be parallel or slightly below hip level.

**Movement:** Place one foot firmly and completely on the step (your heel shouldn't hang off the edge). Drive through your heel and press upward and forward, loading the elevated leg as you bring your other foot onto the platform to meet the working leg. Don't push off or bounce to create momentum with the leg on the

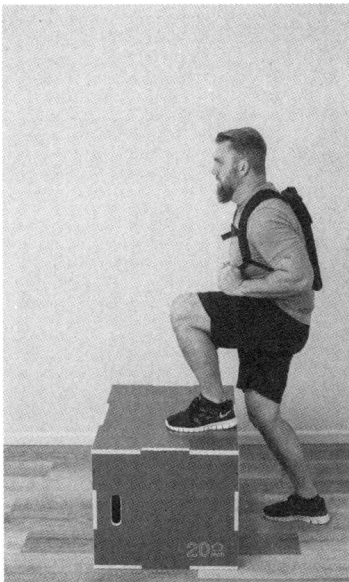

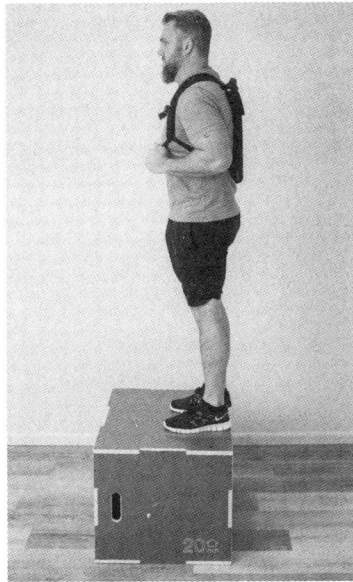

ground. Slowly lower your nonworking leg back to the ground, maintaining smooth, steady control. Repeat all reps on one side before switching legs, or alternate legs with each step-up.

**Make it easier:**
- Use a lower box or step to reduce the range of motion.
- Use only your body weight.
- For extra stability, place your hand on a wall or rail.

**Make it harder:**
- Use a taller box or bench to increase the range of motion.
- Increase the ruck weight or hold on to dumbbells or kettlebells for added resistance.
- After stepping down, immediately step back into a reverse lunge to increase intensity and work both legs.

# MOBILITY WORK

Mobility isn't just about athletic performance. It's critical for maintaining independence as you age. In fact, nearly 15 percent of Americans struggle with walking or climbing stairs, according to the CDC. It's an everyday task we take for granted, but just like muscle, mobility fades if you don't use it.

Harvard Health breaks mobility down into five key components: balance, coordination, range of motion, stamina, and strength.[29] Rucking can improve four of the five elements, but for range of motion, rucking alone isn't enough. That's where stretching and yoga come into play.

## *Stretching*

Think of stretching as more than just a way to cool down after a workout. It's a reset button for increasing range of motion, lengthening tight muscles, and improving posture. So don't make it an afterthought. Regular stretching helps:

**Improve flexibility.** Better range of motion means more agility and fewer restrictions.

**Prevent injuries.** Easing tension in tight muscles and joints reduces stiffness that can lead to strains or other injuries.

**Relieve stress.** Stretching works for your mind, too. It taps in to your parasympathetic nervous system to promote relaxation and reduce tension.

**Boost circulation.** Better blood flow to muscles aids recovery, reduces soreness, and helps you prepare for your next challenge.

New ruckers commonly experience muscle soreness and joint stiffness, and stretching goes a long way in easing that discomfort. Just a few minutes of post-ruck stretching or a dedicated mobility session can make a world of difference, and your body will thank you for it.

## Yoga: Targeted Mobility Exercises

Yoga combines stretching, balance, and mindfulness, making it a fantastic complement to rucking. Many ruckers credit yoga with improving their ruck times and performance. Like rucking and strength training, yoga involves technique. With practice, you'll become familiar with the specific names and flows. If you take a yoga class and fall behind or feel lost, remember that, much like rucking, it's not a competition. You learn as you go.

The exercises in this section aren't exhaustive, instead they serve as a solid starting point to help keep you moving comfortably. You might find it beneficial to use a yoga mat and/or yoga blocks. While neither is required, they can make stretching more comfortable and accessible. A yoga mat provides cushioning, traction, and a clean surface for stretching or mobility work. Look for a mat that's nonslip, moderately thick (4 to 6 mm), and easy to clean. Yoga blocks offer extra support, allowing you to modify poses to suit your current flexibility and ensure safety. A yoga strap is another tool that can help hold positions and extend your reach. In a pinch, you can substitute a towel for a yoga strap or mat, and books or sturdy containers can serve as alternatives to blocks. Regardless of your setup, the following poses can be performed anywhere—at home, outdoors, or after a ruck—whenever you want to rest, reset, or work on your range of motion.

## DOWNWARD DOG

This well-known pose strengthens and lengthens key muscle groups involved in rucking. It targets the hamstrings, calves, shoulders, and upper back while gently elongating the spine and arches of the feet.

**Starting position:** Start in tabletop position (on your hands and knees, with your shoulders over your wrists and hips over your knees). Spread your fingers wide, with your middle finger pointed to the top of your mat and weight distributed evenly from palms to fingertips.

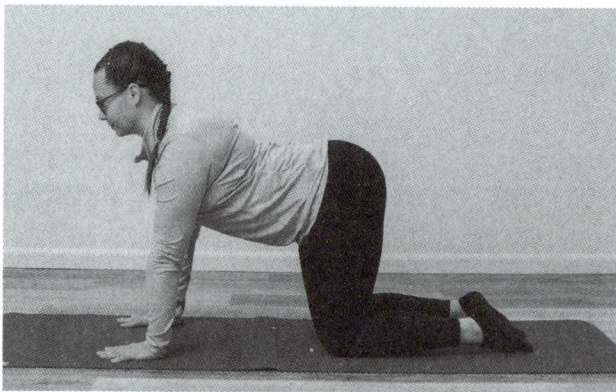

**Movement:** Inhale and tuck your toes. As you exhale, gently lift your knees off the mat and press your hips up and back. Straighten your legs as much as your flexibility allows, keeping a slight bend in your knees and pressing your heels toward the ground. It's OK if they don't touch the mat. Your feet should be hip-width apart, parallel to each other, and facing the front of your mat—not pointing outward. Pull your belly button toward your spine to engage your core muscles and support your lower back. Imagine wrapping your shoulder blades around your ribcage and pressing the floor away from you, creating a straight line from your wrists to your hips and lifting your tailbone to the ceiling. Keep your head between your arms, gazing toward your knees or navel. Take three to five breaths before returning to your hands and knees.

**Make it different:**
- Place your hands or forearms on yoga blocks to change the angle.
- "Walk the dog" by pedaling your feet. Alternate bending one knee while pressing the opposite heel toward the ground, which deepens the stretch into the calves and hamstrings.

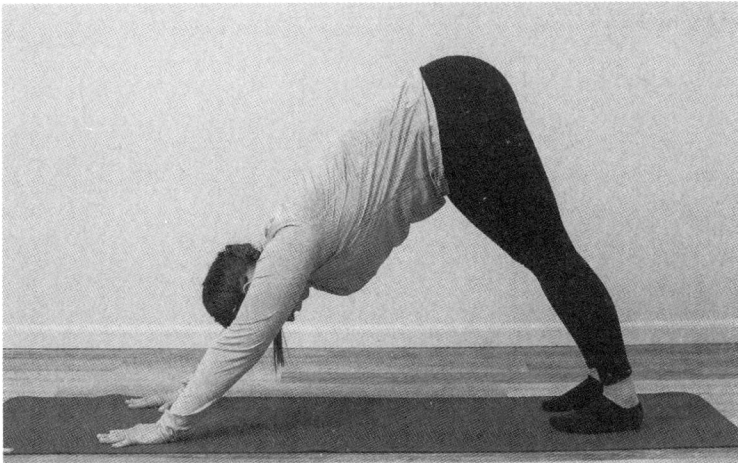

## PIGEON POSE

This popular posture provides a deep stretch for the hips, glutes, and hip flexors. It's especially helpful if you spend long hours sitting, and it improves lower body mobility. If, like me, you have tight hips, you may develop a love-hate relationship with this stretch. It hurts so good but feels so good when you're done! If you have grumpy knees, ease into pigeon pose slowly or skip to the lying Figure Four (page 130), which targets the same muscles.

**Starting position:** Start in tabletop, on hands and knees, or downward dog position, with your hands shoulder-width apart and knees hip-width apart.

**Movement:** Bring your right knee toward your right wrist, lying your leg on the mat. Position your right ankle near your left wrist, adjusting the angle of your shin depending on your flexibility. (The more parallel your shin is to the front of the mat, the deeper the stretch.) Slide your left leg straight back, keeping your hips square to the mat.

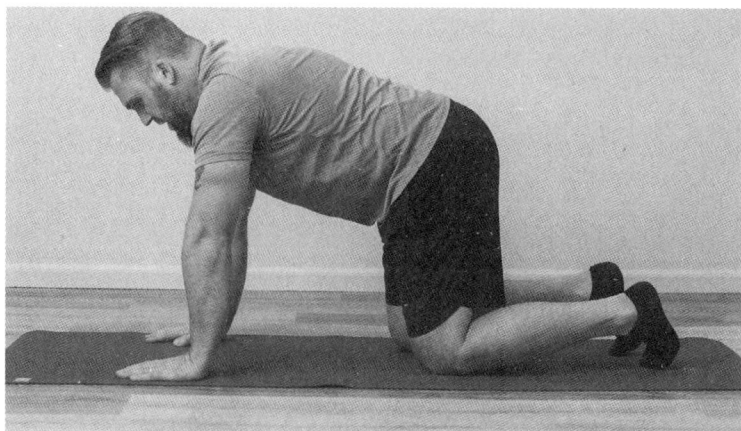

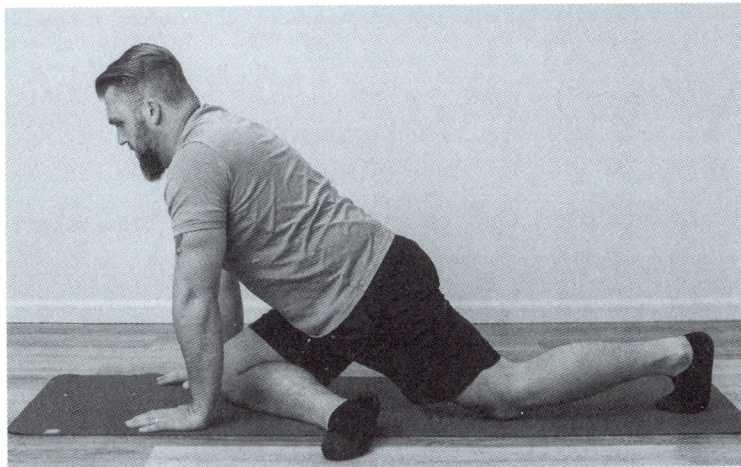

Place your hands on the mat for support or walk them forward, eventually resting your forearms on the ground. Hold for 45 to 60 seconds, releasing the muscles around your hips. Focus on deep breathing, softening any areas of tension and sending your breath to any tight spots, such as your outer glute. When you're ready, gently press back up to tabletop or downward dog and repeat on the left side.

**Make it easier:**
- If your hips feel tight, position the ankle of the bent leg closer to your groin.
- Use props, such as a folded blanket or yoga block under your hip on the bent-leg side, to provide extra support and keep your hips level.
- Place a yoga block under your chest or prop yourself up with blocks until you can do the stretch unsupported.

**Make it harder:** Walk your hands farther forward and rest your chest or forehead on the mat for a deeper stretch.

## CHILD'S POSE

This simple yet powerful yoga pose is commonly used as a resting position. By relaxing tight hips and opening muscles in the back and shoulders, this stretch helps relieve tension that can accumulate from rucking.

**Starting position:** Begin in a kneeling or tabletop position with your knees wider than hip-width apart. Bring your big toes to touch behind you.

**Movement:** Sit your hips back toward your heels, extending your arms in front of you with your palms pressing into the ground. Lower your chest toward the floor, gently resting your forehead on the mat. Imagine wrapping your shoulder blades around your ribcage, taking slow, deep breaths, in through your nose and out through your mouth. Let gravity deepen the stretch with every breath. Hold for as long as you wish.

**Make it easier:** Elevate your torso with a bolster or pillow under your chest.

**Make it harder:** "Thread the needle" by guiding one arm under your chest and across your body to meet the opposite elbow. This movement adds a spinal twist and extra stretch throughout the upper back and shoulders.

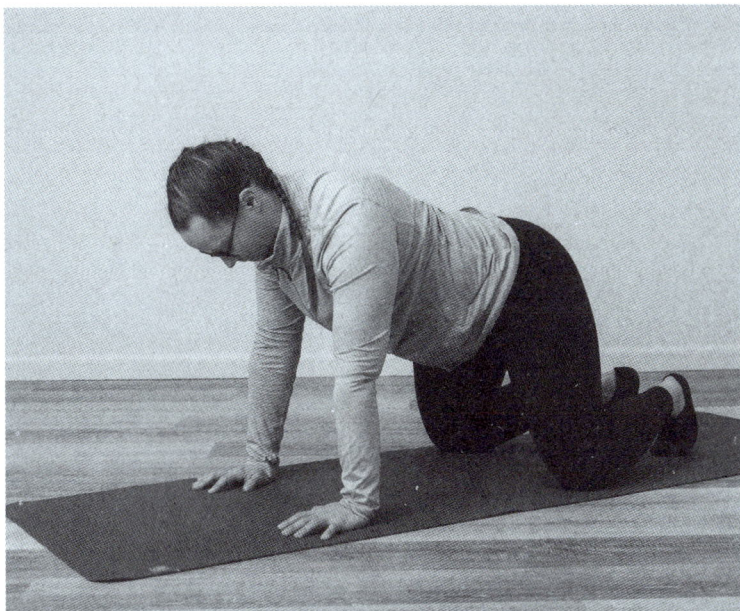

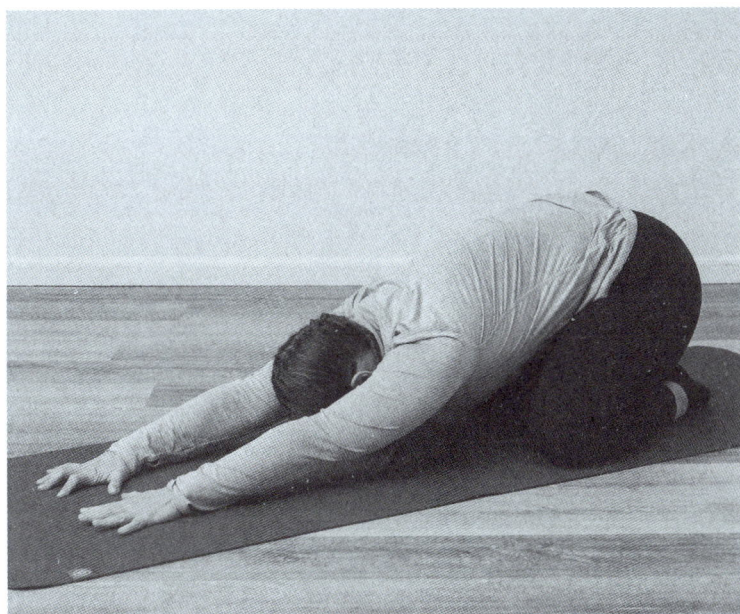

## FIGURE FOUR

This versatile stretch targets the hips, glutes, piriformis, and lower back, and it proves especially beneficial for relieving tightness from prolonged sitting or intense workouts. Use it as an alternative to Pigeon Pose (page 126) to lessen knee strain. You can do it seated, standing, or lying on your back.

**Starting position:** Lie flat on your back on a yoga mat or other comfortable surface. With your knees bent and feet flat on the floor, lift your right leg and place your right ankle on your left thigh, just above the knee. Flex your right foot. Your right leg crosses over your left leg, resembling the number four and giving the stretch its name.

**Movement, lying version:** Reach your hands around your left leg, clasping the back of your leg with both hands and lifting your left foot off the floor. Pull your left thigh toward your chest while keeping your shoulders and head relaxed on the mat. Adjust the intensity by pulling your left thigh closer to your chest. Hold for 30 to 60 seconds, releasing any tension in your hips and glutes. Gently release your grip and switch legs, repeating the stretch on the left side.

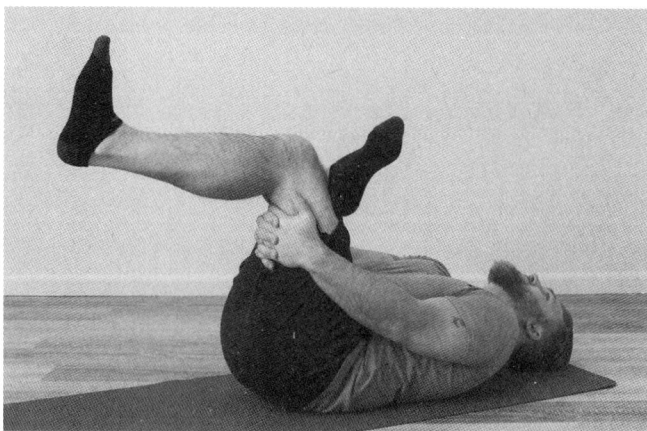

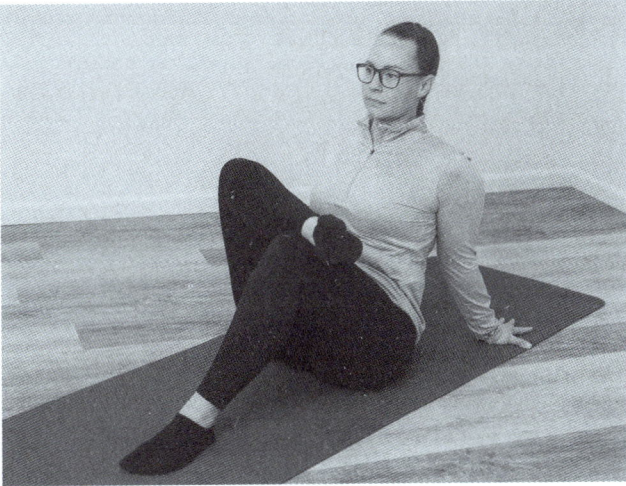

**Movement, seated version:** Keeping your right ankle above your left knee, press yourself onto your forearms, then into a seated position with your arms straight and fingers pointed toward the back of your mat. Adjust the intensity by bringing your upper body closer or farther to your bent leg. Hold the stretch for 30 to 60 seconds before returning to the starting position and repeating on your left side.

**Make it easier:**
- If clasping your thigh feels challenging, loop a yoga strap or towel around the back of your leg. Hold the ends, letting it do the work while keeping your upper body relaxed and pressed tight to the ground.
- Do this stretch seated in a chair. Cross your right ankle over your left thigh, gently pressing your right knee down to increase the intensity of the stretch.

**Make it harder:** Perform this stretch while standing. Cross your right ankle over your left knee and sit back as if there were a chair behind you. Hold on to a sturdy surface for extra support.

## LYING CROSSBODY STRETCH

This is one of my favorite stretches and targets the lower back, glutes, and spine, helping reduce stiffness and improve flexibility. It won't take long to feel the results.

**Starting position:** Lie flat on your back on a yoga mat or comfortable surface. Extend your legs and bring your left knee in, hugging it toward your chest. Keep your right leg extended long.

**Movement:** Use your right hand to guide your left knee across your body, lowering it toward the floor on the right side. Keep your left shoulder grounded and your left arm extended in a T shape. Turn your head to look toward your left hand for an added spinal twist. Relax into the stretch. You should feel a gentle release in your left glute and throughout your spine and chest.

Hold this position for 30 to 60 seconds, breathing deeply and allowing your body to relax with each exhalation. When you're ready, gently bring your knee back to the starting position and repeat the stretch on the opposite side.

**Make it easier:** Place a folded blanket, cushion, or yoga block under the knee you're crossing over.

**Make it harder:**
- Straighten the top leg and aim to touch your foot to the ground for a deeper stretch.
- Experiment with raising the knee of your top leg, feeling the stretch move deeper into your hips and outer glute.

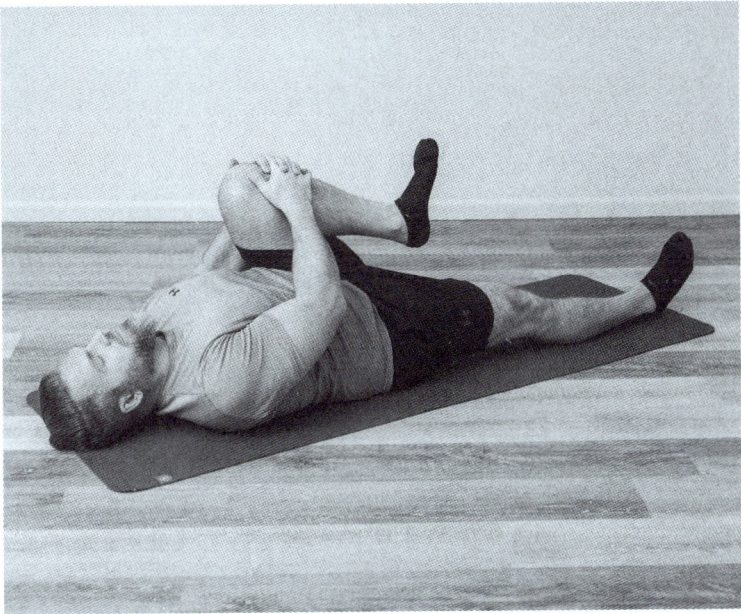

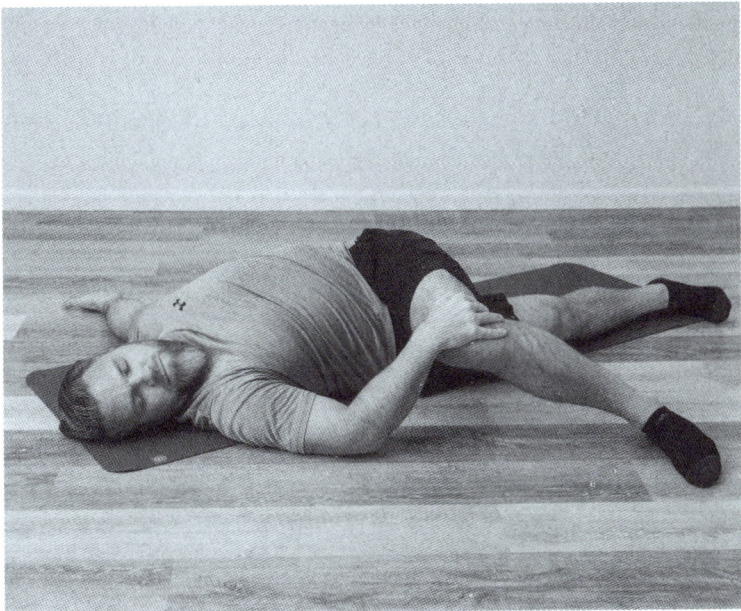

## SEATED 90/90 STRETCH

Another one of my favorites, this stretch helps improve hip mobility and relieve tightness in the glutes and hips. The next time you're binge-watching your favorite show, hop down to the floor and try it.

**Starting position:** On the floor, sit up tall with your legs extended in front of you. Bend your right leg in front of you, creating a 90-degree angle at your knee. If you're on a mat, your shin should run parallel to the front of your mat. Position your left leg to the side, also at a 90-degree angle, with your knee pointing away from your body. Keep your chest lifted and shoulders relaxed.

**Movement:** Place your hands on the ground in front of you and lean forward, over your front leg, to stretch your hip, glute, and lower back. Keep your back straight and legs grounded, maintaining a 90-degree angle at both knees. Hold the stretch for 30 to 60 seconds before returning to the starting position. Repeat on the opposite side.

**Make it easier:** Support yourself using yoga blocks under your hands or sit on a cushion to elevate your hips.

**Make it harder:** Lower your chest closer to the ground, leaning on your forearms or moving your hands farther in front of you to deepen the stretch.

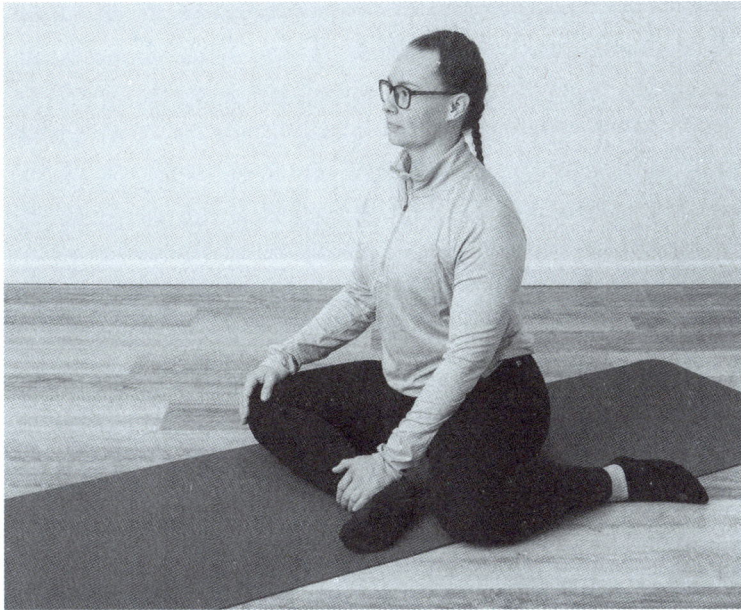

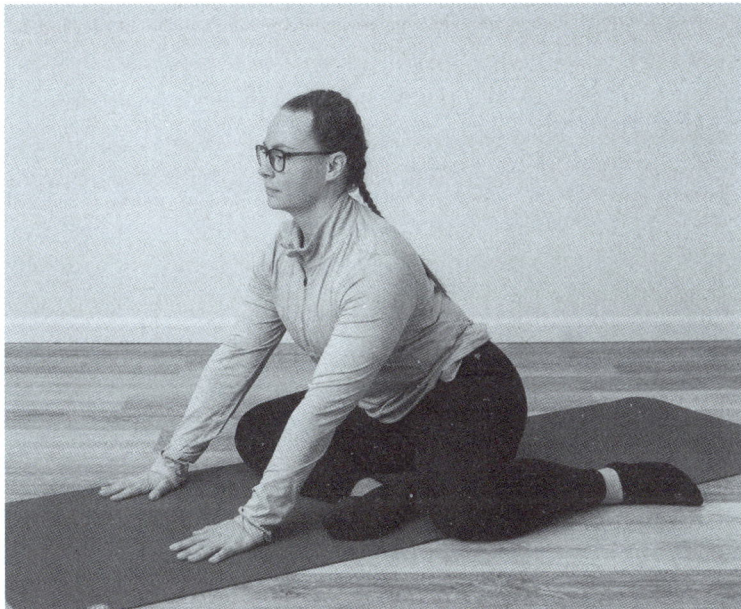

## SEATED HAMSTRING STRETCH

Maybe you remember the sit-and-reach box from grade school PE class—the one where you sat with legs outstretched and reached your fingertips as far as you could? This movement is the grown-up version of that, designed to improve flexibility, ease tightness in the back of the legs, and help you reach your toes without groaning. You can do it seated, standing, or lying on your back. Try all three and see which feels best to you.

**Starting position:** Sit on the floor with your legs extended straight in front of you. Avoid locking your knees and flex your feet so your toes point toward the ceiling. Sit tall, keeping your back straight and shoulders relaxed.

**Movement:** Take a deep breath, and lift and lengthen your spine. Exhale, hinging at your hips, and walk your hands down your thighs, toward your shins and feet. Avoid rounding your back and reaching with your upper body. Instead, imagine tilting the top of your pelvis toward your toes while you lower your chest to your knees. Go as far as you can without hunching your back. Hold for 30 to 60 seconds before returning to the starting position.

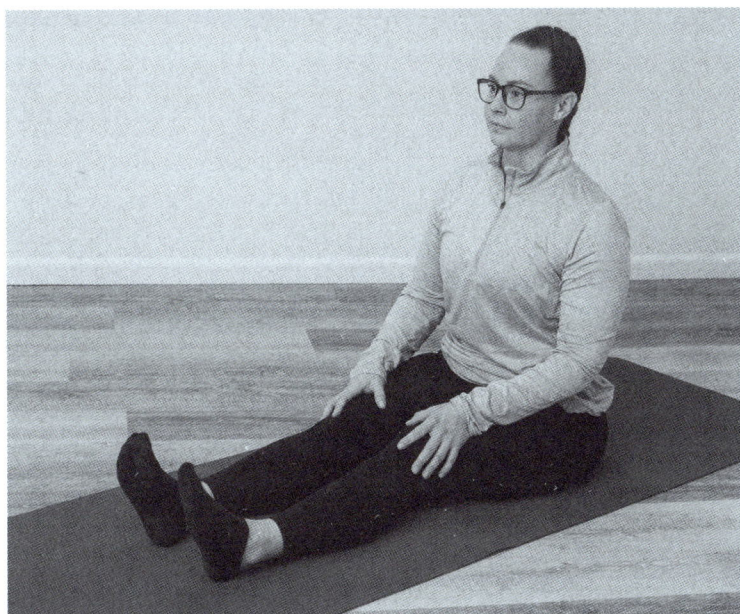

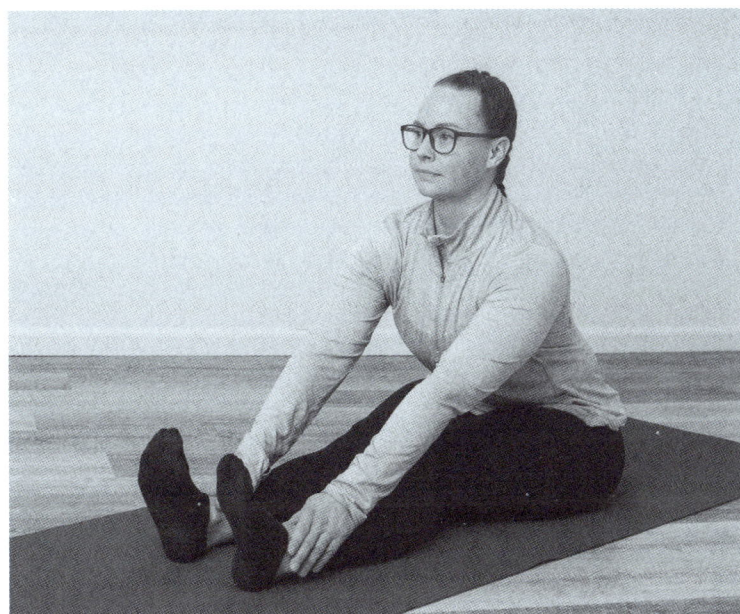

**Variations:** *Figure-four hamstring stretch:* For the starting position, sit with one leg extended straight and the other leg bent with the sole of your foot resting against your inner thigh.

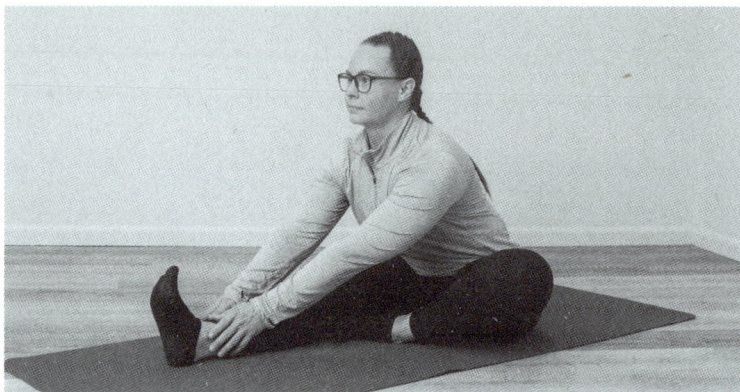

*Standing hamstring stretch:* Stand with your feet hip-width apart. Place one foot on an elevated surface (chair, step, bench), or place your heel on the ground with your toes pointing up. Keep a slight bend in your standing leg and hinge at your hips, reaching toward your toes while maintaining a neutral spine.

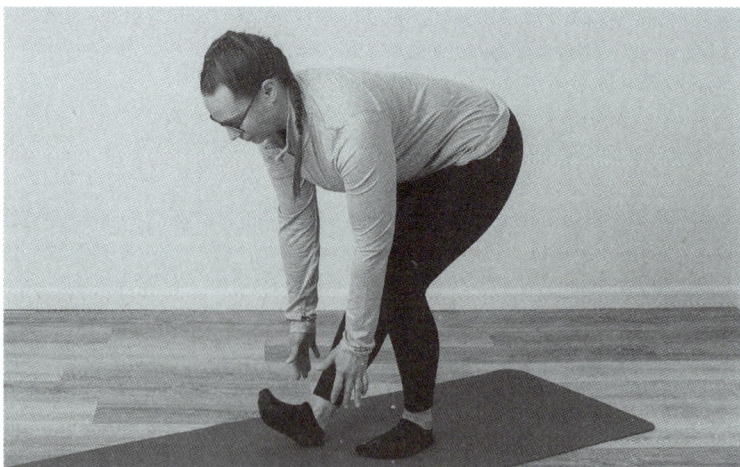

*Lying hamstring stretch with strap:* Lie on your back with one leg extended flat on the ground. Loop a yoga strap, towel, or resistance band around the ball of the opposite foot. Use the strap to pull your leg gently toward your torso while keeping a slight bend in your knee and the other leg planted firmly on the ground.

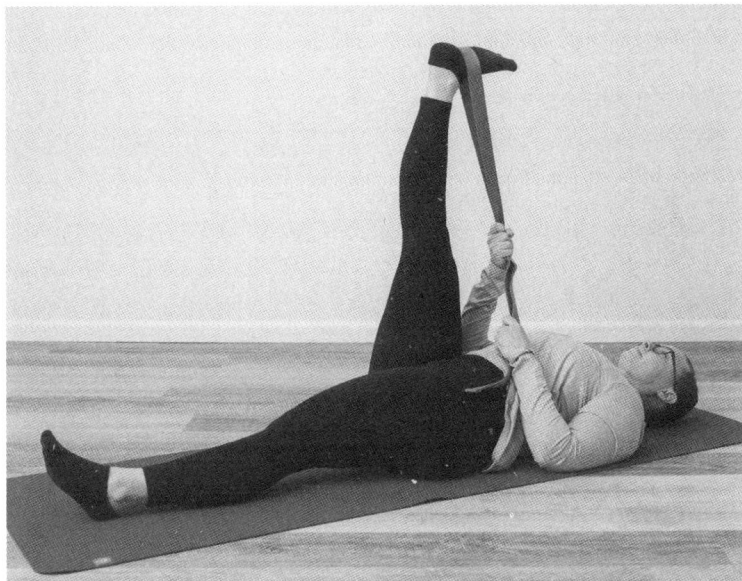

**Make it easier:**
- Keep your knees bent.
- Sit on a cushion or folded blanket to elevate your hips.

**Make it harder:** Hold your feet or toes instead of your shins, keeping your legs as straight as possible.

## STANDING QUAD STRETCH

This stretch is a staple of any well-rounded flexibility routine and targets muscles of the front thigh. Properly stretching the quads improves flexibility and supports knee health. Whether you prefer a classic standing stretch or a more stable lying variation, this exercise suits all fitness levels.

**Starting position:** Stand tall with your feet hip-width apart and core engaged. If needed, hold on to a wall, chair, or sturdy object for support.

**Movement:** Bend your left knee and reach back to grab your left ankle or the top of your foot with your left hand. Keep your knees zipped together, pointing your bent knee toward the ground. Gen-

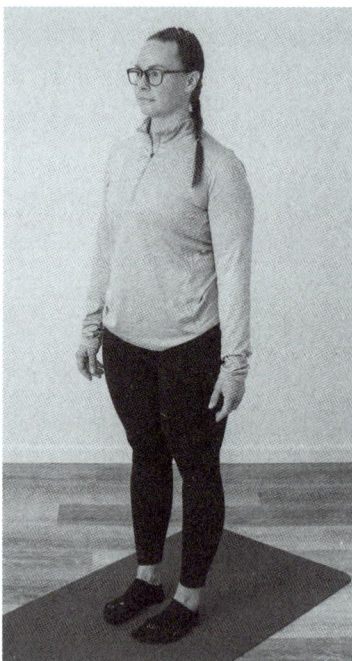

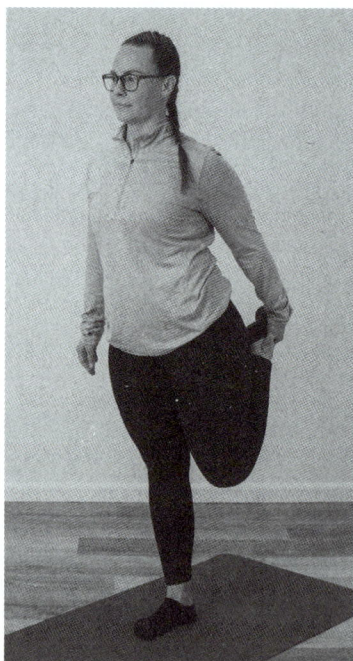

tly pull your ankle toward your butt, pressing your hips forward and squeezing your left glute until you feel a stretch in the front of your thigh. Keep your chest lifted and shoulders down and back. Hold for 30 to 60 seconds, then slowly release your foot toward the ground and switch sides.

**Variations:** *Lying quad stretch:* Lie on your stomach with your legs extended. Rest your forehead on your right forearm. Bring your left foot toward your butt, grabbing your ankle or the top of your foot with your left hand. Pull your foot toward your glute, pressing your pelvis into the floor. Hold for 30 to 60 seconds, then slowly release your foot and switch sides.

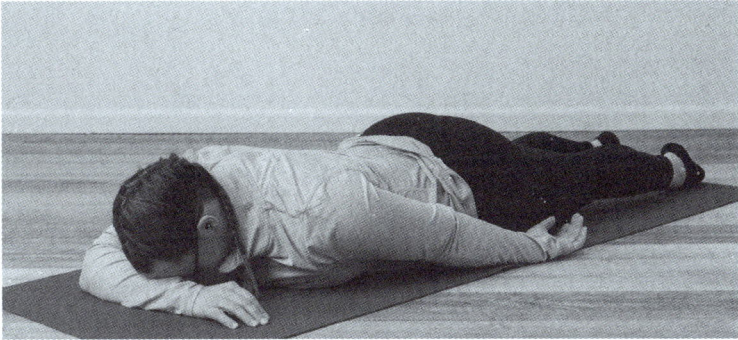

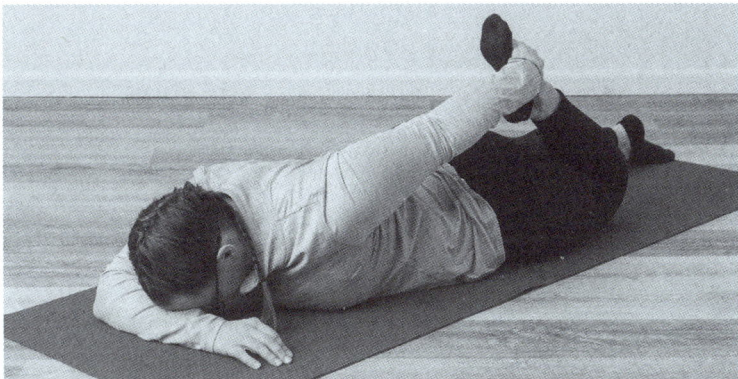

*Side-lying quad stretch:* Lie on your left side with your legs stacked. Extend your left arm and rest your head on your left bicep. Bend your top (right) knee, reaching back to grab your right ankle or foot with your right hand. Keep your thighs aligned as you gently pull your foot toward your glute and press your hips forward. Bend your bottom (left) leg to provide added stability. Hold for 30 to 60 seconds, then switch sides.

**Make it easier:** Use a yoga strap, towel, or resistance band looped around your ankle for extra leverage and support.

**Make it harder:** Perform the movement without holding on to a wall or chair. Engage your core to maintain stability and prevent wobbling.

# FOAM ROLLING

Self-myofascial release, better known as foam rolling, can improve mobility by addressing muscle tightness and breaking up adhesions in the fascia, the connective tissue that wraps around your muscles. No matter how much groaning, wincing, or internal debating, I always feel better and looser after foam rolling. Sometimes what we dread most is what we need most.

Think of foam rolling as a do-it-yourself massage. It's an excellent recovery tool after any intense workout, including rucking. Benefits include:

**Releasing tight muscles.** Rolling over stiff muscles helps them relax and improves flexibility, making it easier to move through a full range of motion.

**Preventing injuries.** By addressing muscle adhesions and imbalances, foam rolling reduces the risk of strains and overuse injuries.

**Accelerating recovery.** Enhanced circulation delivers oxygen and nutrients to muscles while removing waste products, such as lactic acid.

Foam rollers come in various densities, lengths, and textures. Some are smooth, while others have ridges or bumps for deeper pressure. If you're new to foam rolling, start with a medium-density roller and move slowly over each muscle group, spending extra time on tight or tender areas. Aim for one to two minutes per muscle group, ensuring the pressure feels firm but not painful. You might feel some surprise pangs on tight spots. That's where you need it most. My go-to moves target the muscles that take the brunt when rucking: quads, hamstrings, and calves. But let's work our way from the top of the body down.

## SHOULDERS AND BACK

When you're rucking, your shoulders and upper back stabilize the load, making them prone to tightness and soreness. Regularly rolling your shoulders and upper back can reduce muscle tension and stiffness, helping you feel more resilient and ready for your next ruck.

**Starting position:** Sit on the floor with the foam roller behind you, perpendicular to your spine. Lie back so the roller is beneath your upper back, just below your shoulder blades. Cross your arms over your chest or support your head with clasped hands.

**Movement:** Engage your core and lift your hips so your torso is parallel to the ground. Slowly roll from your shoulder blades down to your mid-back, pausing at tight or sore spots. Twist gently from side to side to target different parts of your upper back, shoulders, and lats.

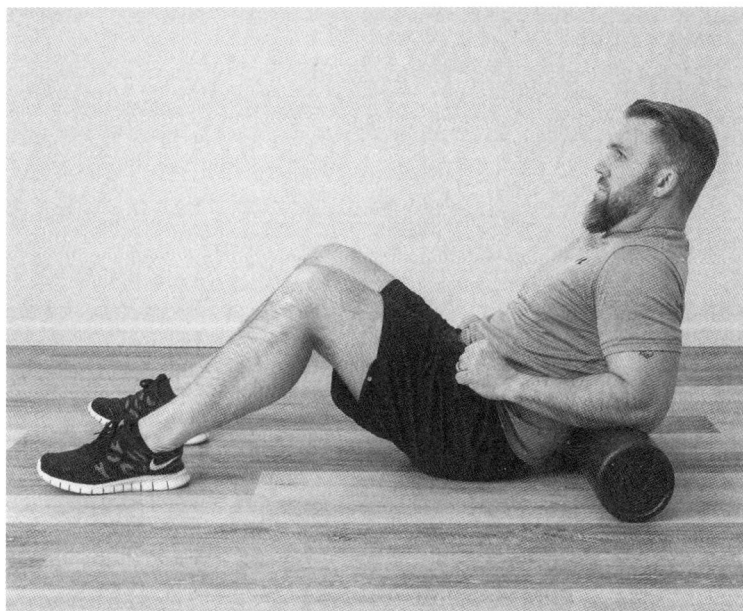

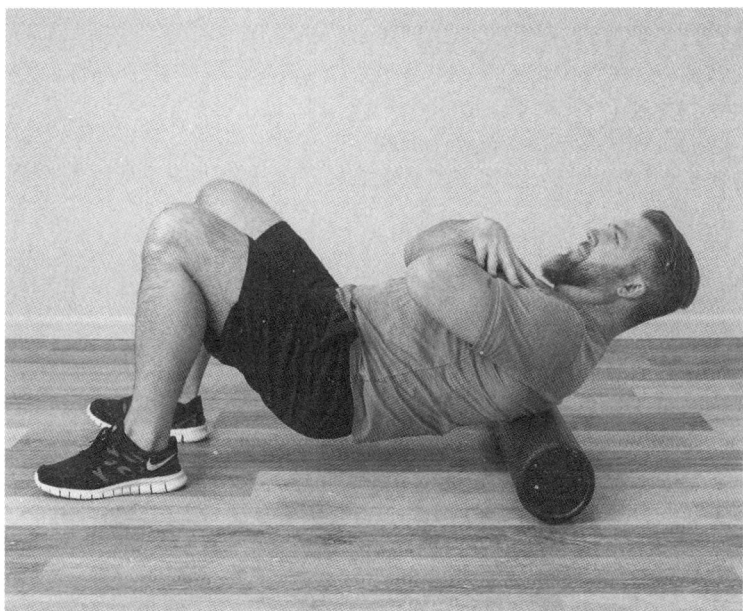

## HAMSTRINGS AND GLUTES

Your glutes and hamstrings can become tight from the repetitive motion of walking and rucking. Foam rolling the posterior chain (back of your body) improves circulation and flexibility, keeping muscles loose and limber, which helps reduce the risk of injury and recover faster.

**Starting position:** Sit on the foam roller, reaching your hands behind you for support. With your feet flat on the ground, bend your knees with your weight supported evenly across all limbs.

**Movement:** Lean to either side, targeting one glute at a time. Slowly roll back and forth from the top of your hip to the bottom of your glute, circling the muscle to hit the inner and outer buttocks. You can also position the foam roller parallel to your leg, rolling the glute from right to left for an even greater release.

Next, move to your hamstrings. Extend your legs and shift your weight to your upper body. Guide the roller from just below your glutes to just above your knees, avoiding direct pressure on the back of the knee. For more pressure, cross one leg over the other and roll one hamstring at a time.

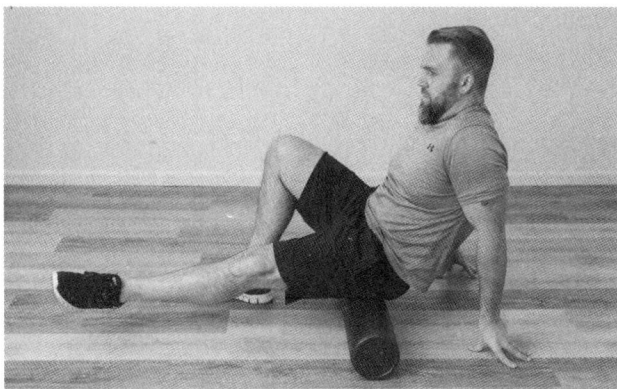

## QUADS

Foam rolling helps loosen up tight quads and reduces tension surrounding your knees to support efficient movement patterns and proper rucking mechanics.

**Starting position:** Lie face down with the foam roller perpendicular to your legs, under one or both thighs. Support yourself with your forearms or hands on the ground.

**Movement:** Use your arms to push your body forward and backward, rolling from the top of your thighs, just below the hip/groin, to above your knees. Never roll over your kneecap. Shift your weight from one side to the other to reach the inner and outer quad.

For more pressure, roll one leg at a time by crossing your ankles behind you and transferring your weight to one side.

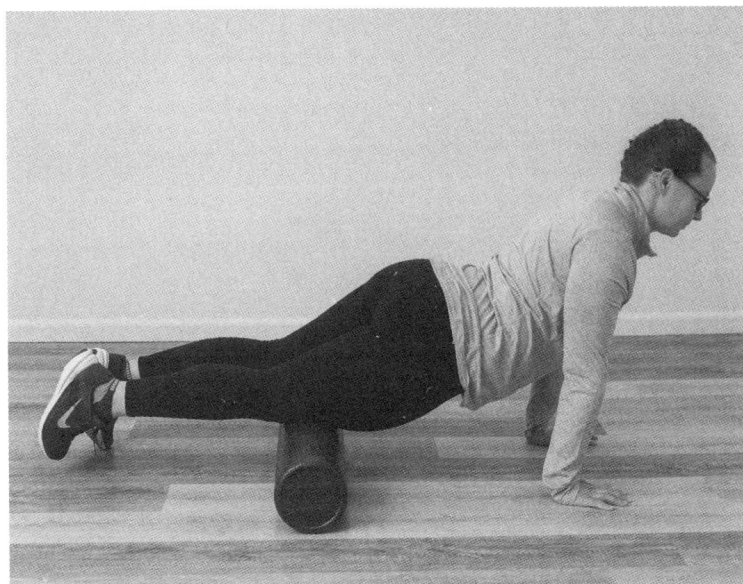

## CALVES

Calves are easy to overlook, but foam rolling keeps these hard-working muscles agile and resilient. You might be surprised by how tight they are until you try these moves, which reduce the risk of cramping, shin splints, and Achilles tendon issues.

**Starting position:** Sit on the floor with your legs extended in front of you. Place the foam roller under the meatiest part of one calf, either perpendicular to your leg or at a 45-degree angle, whichever gives your calf the most contact with the roller. Plant your palms firmly on the floor to support your weight and create a stable base.

**Movement:** Lift your hips off the ground and use your upper body like a pendulum, pushing yourself forward and backward. Roll from the back of your ankle to just below your knee, covering the entire calf muscle. Point your toe and rotate your leg inward

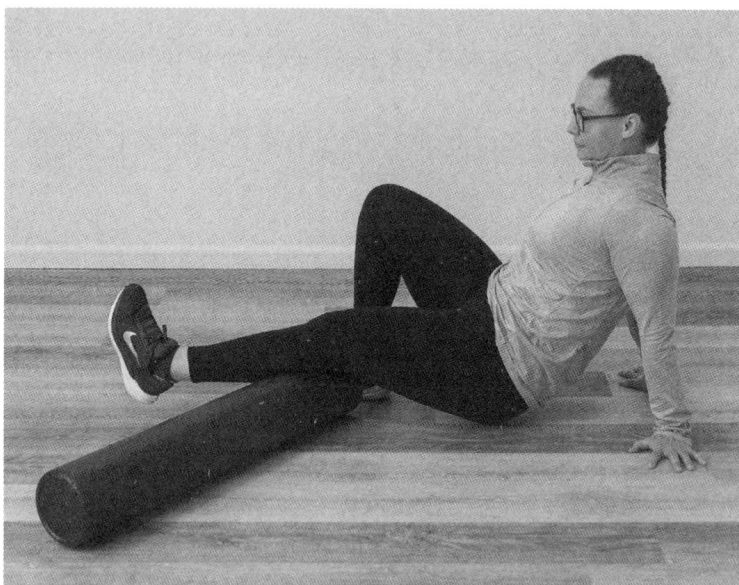

and outward to roll along the sides of your calf, where tension often hides.

For less intensity, remain seated on the ground and focus on one calf at a time. You can also turn the foam roller parallel to your calf and roll it side to side. For more pressure, keep your hips off the ground and cross one leg over the other.

## REMEMBER

► The hardest part of any fitness journey is starting. To avoid getting stuck in the planning process, choose a training program that seems right for you and just begin.

► Sign up for a local rucking race to stay motivated and accountable.

► The *Ruck Fit* training programs are built on three core principles: rucking, strength, and mobility.

► When designing a strength-training routine, try a push-pull-leg (PPL) split to target all major muscle groups throughout the week.

► Compound movements target multiple muscle groups at once, and along with a PPL split, they help facilitate maximum gains in minimal time.

► To enhance recovery and flexibility, complement your rucks and weight training sessions with mobility work, including stretching, yoga, or foam rolling.

# PART THREE

# Fuel Your Resiliency

# 5

## Nutrition Protocols

> There are no solutions,
> only trade-offs.
>
> —LAYNE NORTON, PHD

hate telling people that I'm a registered dietitian. Hearing that, so many people instantly interrogate me about GMOs, the keto diet, or whether a food is "good" or "bad." Even at the best of times, nutrition makes for a messy subject, and it offers countless opportunities for conversations to go off the rails.

Take food manufacturing, for example. Around 15,000 new food products hit grocery store shelves each year. At some companies, food scientists and marketing experts spend up to two years engineering one product.[30] They create highly palatable, highly processed products—often labeled as "low-carb" or "high-protein"—but these claims don't mean they're healthy. The tangled mass of conflicting messages means job security for me, but I'd rather see everyone eat better.

Rather than adding to the noise of diet books and opinions about how to eat "right," this chapter gives you practical, actionable strategies to fuel your rucks and, if it's one of your goals, to shed pounds. Nutrition goes beyond what you eat, and it means fueling yourself with purpose and intention.

# BALANCING BALONEY AND CALORIES

Eating from a specific list of foods or following a detailed meal plan may help lose weight in the short term, sure, but once you deviate, it often leads to weight regain and regret. Sustainable weight loss goes far beyond what we eat and includes how and why we eat. My busy, professional, intelligent clients excel in many areas of life—family, relationships, their career—yet many struggle with their weight. Many of them feel ashamed, desperate for sustainable, lasting change. When we shift their focus from "eat less, move more" to addressing the "how" and "why" of eating, everything begins to transform for them.

Instead of focusing on calories, I teach them to prioritize eating for blood sugar balance and work on their emotional relationship with food. They learn how mindless snacking—even on "healthy" foods such as fruit and 100-calorie snack packs—saps energy, drives cravings, and leads to unwanted weight gain. By swapping calorie counting with continuous glucose monitoring (CGM), they gain real-time insights on how food, stress, exercise, and sleep affect their progress.

This whole-life approach includes setting bedtimes, managing stress, and adding strength training (including rucking) to the formula—and it works. My clients experience fewer cravings, more energy, and less inflammation. They get to the root causes of unwanted weight and improve their relationship with food. They also discover their "worth-it" foods, enjoying their favorite treats guilt-free and without sacrificing results.

Nutrition has become dogmatic, but there is no one right way to eat. It takes trial, error, and practice to find what works for you. And every choice has a trade-off. Want visible abs? You need to commit to clean eating and regular exercise. Hate cooking? Expect to eat the same meals on repeat or pay an arm and a leg for someone else to cook for you. Weigh your options and aim for a net-positive most of the time.

Over the past decade, my views on nutrition have shifted dramatically—often in ways that directly contradict what I was taught in school, like avoiding fat, salt, and red meat. So buckle up for a no-holds-barred conversation about how to leverage nutrition to live a healthy, fulfilling life.

# EXERCISE AND ENERGY BALANCE

You can't out-ruck a bad diet. If moving more is your solution to lose weight, you need a new approach. Exercise is not a way to burn and earn calories, nor is it a punishment for what you ate or plan to eat. You can't outrun a super-sized muffin or save calories for a night out.

Your body isn't a closed system, which means "calories in, calories out" doesn't work as a foolproof tool for weight management. Not all calories are created equal, and their quality matters. For instance, 100 calories of broccoli impact your blood sugar and hunger hormones differently than 100 calories of pretzels. Broccoli contains more fiber, nutrients, and volume, which naturally triggers the release of satiating hormones such as GLP-1, the peptide found in popular weight loss medications.

On top of that, the calories you burn extend far beyond exercise. It takes a *crazy* amount of energy to build and repair body tissues, breathe, and even think. The brain, for example, makes up just 2 percent of body weight, yet it accounts for about 20 percent of daily calorie expenditure.[31] Daily biological maintenance, better known as resting energy expenditure (REE), accounts for roughly two-thirds of your daily calorie burn. A 40-year-old woman who stands 5 feet 5 inches tall and weighs 175 pounds has an REE of approximately 1,500 calories. She burns that much every day *without* even getting out of bed! Exercise aside, you are likely burning more calories than you think. The energy required to digest food and transport nutrients where they need to go represents about a tenth of your daily calorie burn. Physical activity is the most variable factor, making up about 25 percent of your daily calorie expenditure.[32]

Movement might not make up most of your daily burn, but it's still essential. Exercise helps maintain lean muscle mass, the most metabolically active tissue in your body. More lean muscle means more calories burned at rest. If you love to eat, having more lean body mass means you can eat more while still losing or maintaining your weight.

Another concept I teach my clients is how to prioritize fat loss over weight loss. When the number on the scale drops, it reflects changes in water weight, fat, *and* muscle. If your fitness routine doesn't include regular physical activity, 20 to 40 percent of "weight" loss can come from losing muscle. To maintain your metabolism, you need to lose fat and preserve or build muscle. To do both at the same time (which is no easy task), two habits are a must: eating enough protein and resistance training.

Calories matter, especially if your goal is fat loss, but my goal is to help you focus on smart, long-term strategies. If you've tried to lose weight by slashing your calorie intake, increasing exercise, or both, only to experience brain fog, fatigue, and stalled results, your willpower isn't the problem; your approach is. Instead of obsessing over calorie count, you must focus on calorie *quality*. When you make choices that support stable blood sugar, you won't have to white-knuckle your way through stubborn cravings. You'll have the energy to cook *and* exercise. You'll sleep better, amplifying your mood and overall quality of life. Weight loss becomes a by-product of feeling better from the inside out.

# WHAT TO EAT

Food is made up of three macronutrients: protein, fat, and carbohydrates. These are the big nutrients that provide calories. Micronutrients don't contribute calories but do supply essential vitamins and minerals, including calcium, vitamin D, iron, and more. Protein and carbohydrates each provide 4 calories per gram, and fat supplies 9 calories per gram. While fat is more calorie-dense, it's not a bad thing.

Most foods contain a mix of macronutrients, but for simplicity's sake, we categorize them based on their predominant makeup. For example, a cashew is roughly 70 percent fat, 20 percent carbohydrates, and 10 percent protein. Since fat is the prominent macronutrient, cashews are considered a good source of fat rather than carbs or protein. A grilled chicken breast contains 80 percent protein, 20 percent fat, and no carbs. It's not purely protein, but we still classify it as a protein source. As you can see, food isn't black and white, so your view of it shouldn't be either.

## *Protein*

More than 40 percent of body protein exists in muscle, 25 percent in internal organs, and the remaining 35 percent in skin and blood. Dietary protein plays a critical role in building and repairing these tissues. It supports a healthy immune system and helps produce enzymes and hormones, the body's chemical messengers. Protein also helps regulate appetite in two ways by promoting fullness and decreasing hunger.

Much like the beads of a necklace, amino acids tether together to form proteins. (We must discuss amino acids to understand the differences between animal and plant proteins, so bear with me.) More than 500 amino acids exist in nature, but only 20 make up dietary protein and the human genome. Nine of these are "essential," meaning you need to consume them in food or sup-plements. Your body can make the 11 nonessential amino acids on its own.

Fish, poultry, eggs, meat, and dairy contain all 20 dietary amino acids, including all nine of the essentials. Plant-based pro-teins, such as beans, grains, nuts, and seeds classify as "incom-plete" since they lack one or more of the nine essential amino acids. Plant protein is also less digestible than animal protein, by about 15 percent. Eggs, for example, are 97 percent digestible, whereas cooked split peas are roughly 70 percent digestible. This math can prove tricky on a nutrition label. For example, one large egg has 6 grams of protein, and ½ cup of cooked split peas has 8 grams of protein. Split peas seem like the clear choice in terms of protein, but after accounting for digestibility, the egg comes in first with 6 grams versus 5.5 grams in the split peas.

That doesn't make plant protein inferior in any way, though. It simply means if you prefer plant-based protein, you need to be intentional and consume *more* protein to make up the difference. Plant-based foods certainly deserve a spot on your plate and pro-vide lots of healthy nutrients, including fiber for gut health and phytochemicals to help combat oxidative stress.

Quality aside, let's talk quantity. Unlike carbs and fat, your body doesn't store protein. That's why it's important to eat enough of it, ideally spread across your day. Your liver is the gatekeeper and keeps tabs on your body's pool of amino acids, monitoring what you eat and the constant turnover of tissue. Your body renews bone tissue every 10 years, for example, while softer tissues such as organs and muscle turn over every six weeks. It doesn't happen all at once, but this constant renovation requires an enormous amount of energy and amino acids , accounting for 10 to 25 per-cent of REE.[33]

So how much protein do you need? For adults, the recom-mended dietary allowance (RDA) for protein is 0.8 grams per kilogram of body weight, or 0.36 grams per pound. That's the minimum amount to avoid deficiency, though, not to live optimally. Many health experts consider the RDA insufficient.

Muscle health expert Dr. Gabrielle Lyon and the International Protein Board (iPB) suggest a protein intake of nearly twice the RDA. The iPB recommends 1.1 to 1.8 grams per kilogram (0.5 to 0.8 gram per pound) for general fitness, weight loss, and healthy aging. For muscle growth and advanced sport, they suggest 1.8 to 2.2 grams per kilogram (0.8 to 1.0 grams per pound). Following those guidelines, a 200-pound person should aim for 100 to 200 grams of protein per day, the lower end for general health and the higher end for muscle growth. For a protein range tailored to your target weight and goals, visit the iPB website (internationalproteinboard.org) and use their free online calculator.[34]

To estimate how much protein you're eating, log your meals with an app such as Cronometer, Lose It!, or Carb Manager to see how your weekly intake compares to the preceding recommendations. For some people, the suggested ranges can feel like a far cry from how much protein they're eating now, but hitting that target doesn't have to be complicated. Here's how to make it easier:

**Start your day with a high-protein meal.** To preserve or put on muscle, consume at least 30 grams of high-quality protein with your first meal, whether it's breakfast or lunch. This quantity specifically sparks muscle growth.[35] Examples include a whey protein shake, Greek yogurt parfait, or an omelet with cheese and/or meat.

**Distribute protein throughout the day.** Quarter your goal and spread it across three meals and a snack. For a 200-pound person focusing on general health, that means 25 grams per meal or snack.

**Keep convenient options on hand.** Stock up on hard-boiled eggs, protein bars and shakes, string cheese, and/or jerky for ready-to-eat options.

**Batch-cook high-protein foods.** Proteins take the most time to prepare. If you're cooking chicken or ground beef, make extra so you have plenty of leftovers.

Experiment with these tips to find what works best for you. Meaningful change doesn't happen overnight, so gradually modify your protein intake from week to week until you reach your goal. At the end of this section (page 165), you'll find an easy-to-read food list that showcases each macronutrient and suggested foods. You can find a printable PDF on my website at kaylagirgenrd.com.

## Fat

For decades, the sugar industry intentionally misled us by portraying fat as the enemy, associating it with heart disease and the false logic that "fat makes you fat." Fat *doesn't* make you fat; excess calories do. But because fat is the most calorie-dense macronutrient, people shunned it in favor of low-fat and fat-free products that surged in popularity starting in the 1980s.

Food manufacturers replaced fat with sugar and refined carbs to maintain taste and flavor. In doing so, they stripped away the satiating quality fat provides, making people who ate these new products more prone to overeat. To replicate the mouthfeel and satisfaction of fat, it requires a cocktail of carb-derived fillers and artificial ingredients. On your next trip to the grocery store, compare the ingredients list of a full-fat product to its fat-free counterpart. The fat-free list probably runs much longer.

More than just a source of flavor or calories, fat represents an indispensable building block for numerous critical processes in the body, such as:

**Vitamin absorption:** Certain vitamins (A, D, E, K) are fat-soluble, meaning, without dietary fat, your body can't access the benefits of these essential nutrients. For maximum absorption, take your multivitamin or vitamin D supplement with a meal containing fat.

**Hormone production:** Dietary fat plays a key role in the synthesis of chemical messengers, influencing everything from metabolism to mood to sexual health and more.

**Cellular structure:** Fat and cholesterol form the foundation of cell membranes. The brain consists of about 60 percent fat, making this macronutrient critical for cognitive function and mental clarity.[36]

**Inflammation control:** Some fats (trans fats) promote inflammation, while others like omega-3 fatty acids help reduce chronic inflammation linked to heart disease, arthritis, cognitive decline, and other conditions.[33]

**Blood sugar regulation:** Healthy fats, when eaten with carbohydrates, slow glucose absorption, helping minimize blood sugar spikes and crashes. Steadier blood sugar levels reduce cravings and improve energy throughout the day.

Not all fats are created equal, and some prove necessary for optimal health. As with amino acids, "essential" fatty acids must come from dietary sources since the body can't make them on its own. These include:

**Omega-3 fatty acids** in fatty fish such as salmon, mackerel, and sardines, as well as plant sources including flaxseeds, chia seeds, and walnuts.

**Omega-6 fatty acids** in vegetable oils, nuts, and seeds.

The Standard American Diet (appropriately nicknamed "SAD") is inundated with omega-6 fats, thanks to the use of cheap, highly processed vegetable oils. Most people meet their omega-6 needs without trying, so maintaining a healthy ratio of the two typically means prioritizing omega-3-rich foods.

Lastly, without getting too technical, a quick overview of saturated and unsaturated fats is in order to help you make healthy, informed food choices:

**Saturated Fats:** Usually solid at room temperature; commonly found in coconut, palm oil, full-fat dairy, and red meat; traditionally vilified for raising LDL ("bad") cholesterol.

**Unsaturated Fats:** Often liquid at room temperature; monounsaturated fatty acids (MUFAs), commonly found in avocados, nuts, and olives, can reduce LDL cholesterol while increasing HDL ("good") cholesterol; polyunsaturated fatty acids (PUFAs), commonly found in walnuts, flaxseeds, sunflower oil, and fatty fish, reduce inflammation, lower the risk of heart disease, and support overall health.

**Trans Fats:** Unsaturated fats turned into saturated fats through hydrogenation; commonly found in commercial baked goods, deep-fried foods, margarine, nondairy creamer, and shortening; increase LDL cholesterol and lower HDL cholesterol.

## Carbohydrates

The word itself conjures images of highly processed foods such as bread, baked goods, candy, crackers, and pretzels. But carbs encompass a broad range of foods, including nutrient-dense vegetables, beans, fruits, and dairy. Rather than thinking of carbs as good or bad, imagine a "carb continuum," with broccoli on one end and a slice of white bread on the other. Both foods primarily consist of carbs, but each impacts the body differently.

Carbs cause a lot of debate, with advocates across the spectrum—high-carb, low-carb, no-carb, and all points in between. Age, overall health, body composition, activity level, gut health, and more affect individual carb tolerance. What works for one person may not work for another, underscoring the importance of personalized nutrition.

Of the macronutrients, carbs have the most direct, immediate effect on blood sugar. "Fast" carbs, including sugar and processed grains, digest quickly, causing a rapid blood sugar spike. "Slow" carbs, such as vegetables and legumes, lead to a more gradual rise in blood sugar. The difference often lies in fiber content. The human body can't digest fiber, a type of carbohydrate classified as soluble or insoluble, depending on whether it dissolves in water. Soluble fiber—in beans, oats, fruits, and veggies—combines with water to form a gel-like substance that slows digestion and helps regulate blood sugar and cholesterol. Insoluble fiber—from whole grains, nuts, seeds, and vegetables—doesn't dissolve in water, adding bulk to the stool, helping food pass more quickly through the digestive system, and preventing constipation.[33] Both kinds of fiber promote digestive health, especially when consumed in whole foods (vegetables, beans) rather than supplements (fiber powder) for reasons that science doesn't fully understand yet.

Unlike fat and protein, there are no "essential" carbohydrates, meaning the human body doesn't require carbs to sustain life. They're still necessary for energy and nutrients, but not eating them won't kill you.

If you're curious about how carbs affect you, continuous glucose monitoring (CGM) can reveal your response to certain foods. Worn on the back of the upper arm or abdomen, a CGM sensor tracks blood sugar in real time. This insight offers a unique window into how fasting, specific foods, meal combinations, exercise, and sleep impact the body. Two people might eat the same bowl of oatmeal but have two completely different blood sugar responses. One person might see a steady rise and fall in glucose, whereas the other might experience a sharp spike and crash. This kind of variation depends on insulin sensitivity, microbiome diversity, meal composition—whether protein or fat was consumed with the carbs—and more. (The next section goes into more detail about food pairing.) Using a CGM allows you to identify patterns and make informed dietary decisions. You can experiment with different foods, portion sizes, and meal combinations to optimize your blood sugar response. Over time, this data can help you:

**Reduce energy crashes** by avoiding the post-meal slump that often follows a blood sugar spike and crash.

**Improve athletic performance** by learning which carb sources fuel workouts without causing sluggishness.

**Support weight management** by reducing cravings and overeating, making it easier to stick to your goals.

**Enhance long-term health** by reducing inflammation and the risk of chronic conditions such as diabetes and heart disease.

CGM empowers you with actionable data instead of guesswork or one-size-fits-all dietary advice. As a personalized tool, it can prove invaluable for fine-tuning your diet, balancing blood sugar, and feeling your best. After all, the goal isn't to fear carbs or eliminate them altogether, but to understand and optimize how they can work for you. To eat better, incorporate more of the following blood sugar–friendly foods into your diet.

| Protein | Fat | Slow Carbs | |
|---|---|---|---|
| bacon | almonds | artichokes | lemons |
| beef | avocado | arugula | lentils |
| bison | avocado oil | asparagus | lettuce |
| chicken | Brazil nuts | bamboo shoots | limes |
| cod | butter | bean sprouts | mushrooms |
| collagen | cashews | beans | okra |
| (powder) | cheese | beets | onions |
| cottage cheese | chestnuts | bell peppers | parsnips |
| crab | chia seeds | blackberries | peas |
| eggs | coconut | blueberries | peppers |
| game meats | coconut milk | bok choy | pickles |
| Greek yogurt | coconut oil | broccoli | plums |
| halibut | dark chocolate | Brussels sprouts | pumpkin |
| lamb | flaxseed | butternut squash | radishes |
| pork | ghee | cabbage | raspberries |
| salmon | hazelnuts | carrots | rhubarb |
| sausage | heavy cream | cauliflower | romaine |
| scallops | hemp hearts | celery | rutabagas |
| seafood | hummus | chickpeas | salad greens |
| shrimp | macadamia | clementines | sauerkraut |
| tempeh | nuts | collard greens | seaweed |
| tilapia | mayonnaise | cranberries | snap peas |
| tofu | (avocado oil) | cucumbers | snow peas |
| tuna | MCT oil | daikon | spinach |
| turkey | nut butter | edamame | sprouts |
| whey protein | olives | eggplants | squash |
| venison | olive oil | fennel | strawberries |
| | pecans | green beans | Swiss chard |
| | pine nuts | hearts of palm | tomatillos |
| | pistachios | hot peppers | tomatoes |
| | pumpkin seeds | jicama | turnips |
| | sesame seeds | kale | water chestnuts |
| | sour cream | kimchi | zucchini |
| | sunflower seeds | kohlrabi | |
| | walnuts | leeks | |

To fuel your workouts and recovery, eat whole-food carbs: starchy vegetables (potatoes, sweet potatoes, corn, parsnips), fruit (any kind), oats (steel cut or rolled), quinoa, or any variety of rice. On their own, these foods will raise your blood sugar more than slow carbs, but with some clever pairing, they don't have to. For some people, strategically eating these nutrient-dense, carb-rich options may contribute to better mood, improved sleep, and a greater ability to stick with a nutrition plan over time.

# HOW TO EAT

Meal timing and the order you eat macronutrients can have a significant impact on blood glucose. Why does that matter? Blood sugar stability helps improve energy, mood, and mental clarity while reducing inflammation and the risk of chronic diseases such as diabetes and heart disease. When you have more energy and fewer cravings, it's easier to exercise, cook healthy meals, and tackle your to-do list. Successful weight loss becomes a by-product of leveling out your blood sugar. Not to mention, you *feel* better too.

You don't need to avoid blood sugar spikes altogether, though. Glucose spikes are a normal response to eating and other inputs. Stress, lack of sleep, and exercise can elevate blood sugar, too. The goal is to minimize the frequency and height of the spikes, creating smoother, steadier curves and reducing overall glucose variability.

After you eat, your blood sugar naturally rises, and your pancreas releases insulin, which shuttles glucose from the bloodstream into your cells, where it becomes chemical energy. Without insulin, sugar in the blood would stay elevated. For most people, the issue isn't a lack of insulin but too much of it. Excess insulin in the bloodstream can lead to insulin resistance and metabolic disease. Limiting blood sugar spikes reduces unwanted insulin surges. Each macronutrient impacts blood glucose differently, as illustrated by the following chart.

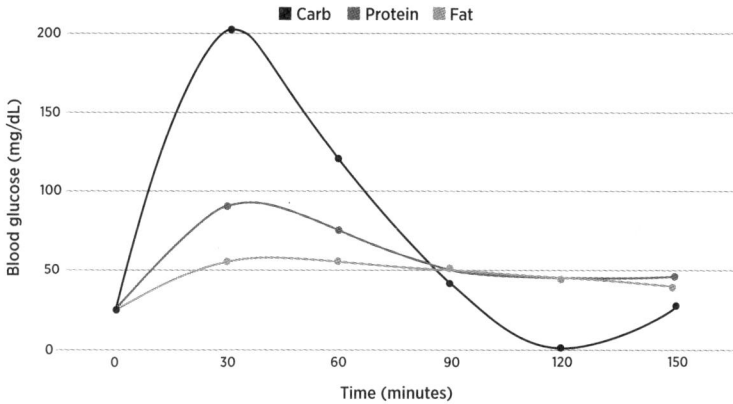

Typical impact of macronutrients on blood sugar over time.

Protein and fat barely nudge blood sugar. Carbs, however, cause a sharp rise and drop in blood sugar, sometimes with a rebound below baseline levels. This can lead to hypoglycemia, with uncomfortable symptoms such as fatigue, sweating, dizziness, nausea, anxiety, headache, intense hunger, rapid heart rate, blurred vision, and, in extreme cases, loss of consciousness. For some individuals, even "healthy" carbs—such as fruit, yogurt, and whole grains—can have suboptimal effects on blood sugar. To avoid massive spikes and feel your best:

**Pair carbs with protein, fat, and/or fiber.** When eaten alone, carbs digest quickly and spike blood sugar. To buffer these spikes, pair carbs with protein, healthy fat, or fiber to slow digestion. For example, enjoy an apple with a slice of your favorite cheese, or top a slice of toast with avocado.

**Frontload carbs early in the day.** Your body tolerates carbs better in the morning when it's more insulin sensitive.

**Consume vinegar before meals.** Drink a tablespoon of vinegar diluted in water to increase insulin sensitivity before a carby meal. Lots of people like apple cider vinegar, but any vinegar works. Rinse your mouth afterward to save your tooth enamel.

**Eat carbs last.** Eating protein and vegetables before carbs can reduce post-meal blood sugar spikes by up to 50 percent.[37] Start with a salad or protein and finish with potatoes, rice, or other starches.

**Move after meals.** Walking or rucking after a meal reduces blood sugar spikes by up to 40 percent because working muscles help clear glucose from the bloodstream without using insulin. Just 10 to 20 minutes will do it.

**Make "resistant" starches.** Cooking and cooling starchy foods like rice, potatoes, and pasta create "resistant" starches, which act more like fiber and slow digestion. For best results, refrigerate cooked starches overnight. Reheat leftovers and still reap the benefits!

Carbs are not the enemy. With these strategies, you can enjoy your favorite foods without sacrificing results.

## WHY WE EAT

We eat for many reasons, hunger among them. But habits and emotions have a stronger influence on our food choices than we like to admit. Years of working with clients—plus my own ups and downs with food—have shown me the power of doing the inner work, like examining habits and beliefs around food, challenging all-or-nothing thinking, and recognizing emotional triggers that lead to snacking or overeating.

Eating is about more than just survival. Food weaves into the fabric of our lives. We eat to celebrate, connect, soothe, and cope. When we're happy, we eat to keep the good feelings going; and the reverse is true when we eat to soothe boredom, stress, or discomfort. With emotional eating, food becomes a crutch to distract, numb, or fill a void. But this temporary relief often ends in guilt or shame, creating a self-reinforcing, vicious cycle. For example, if you snack because you're stressed about a work deadline, or if you struggle with nighttime eating as a way to "relax," you may need to explore healthier coping strategies. We can't lay off food cold turkey (like we can with other vices like scrolling social media or drinking alcohol), so we have to learn to get along with it.

Habits matter just as much as emotions. Take, for instance, snacking while watching TV. Perhaps your kid or partner is eating, and you feel left out. Another example is the parental ritual of finishing your kids' leftovers to avoid wasting food. These small behaviors sneak quietly into your daily routines, disconnecting you from your body's natural cues for hunger and fullness.

It's not easy to transform your relationship with food. It requires time, patience, and effort, but it's absolutely possible. It starts with a willingness to explore new mindsets and strategies. A colleague once likened the process of changing a habit to treading a new path in a field. At first, the ground is overgrown and unbroken. It takes more effort at the beginning and might require some serious bushwhacking. But with consistent effort, you can stomp, walk, and eventually stroll until the path is smooth. Retraining your brain is no different. To help uncover why you eat, use these strategies to begin peeling the onion of your food habits and behaviors.

**Identify your triggers.** Keep a food journal, not to log calories, but to track how you feel and what you eat. Recognizing patterns can help pinpoint specific emotions, people, situations, or times of day that lead to emotional eating.

**Build a stress-relief tool kit.** Replace food as a coping mechanism with healthier outlets, such as walking, journaling, deep breathing, or talking to a friend. These activities can help process emotions without turning to food.

**Pause before eating.** When the desire to eat strikes, take a moment to ask yourself: *Am I physically hungry, or am I trying to soothe an emotion or reinforce a habit?* Even a short pause can help break the automatic tendency to eat.

**Practice self-compassion.** Emotional eating often conjures up feelings of failure, so remind yourself that this behavior is perfectly normal. When you catch yourself eating out of emotion or habit, treat each occurrence as a learning opportunity instead of a setback to help break the cycle.

**Follow a routine.** Consistent meal and snack times help stabilize blood sugar, making it easier to respond to hunger and cravings rationally rather than emotionally.

**Seek support.** If emotional eating has deep roots in past experiences or current stressors, a therapist, dietitian, or coach can help you address these causes with personalized tactics.

## FUEL YOUR FITNESS ROUTINE

Your body needs sufficient fuel to power through workouts, especially lengthy or intense rucking sessions. As a dietitian, a top question I'm asked is, "How should I fuel my workouts?" Most people are surprised to learn that workouts under an hour usually don't require anything special, as long as you're meeting your daily nutrition needs, especially protein and fluids. For longer or more demanding workouts, proper fueling becomes essential to sustain energy, boost endurance, and support recovery.

Use the following to create a fueling plan tailored to your

needs. This section breaks down fueling into three essential parts: pre-workout, intra-workout, and post-workout.

## Pre-Workout: Setting the Stage

Fueling before a workout requires trial and error. Some people feel energized with a light snack beforehand, whereas others perform better on an empty stomach. What works best for you depends on your preferences, how your body responds, and the timing.

If you exercise right after you wake up, you might not have time for a full meal. In that case, a quick, light snack can provide a boost without weighing you down. If you exercise later in the day or one to two hours after a meal, you might not need to think about pre-workout fuel at all. Either way, these general guidelines can help you prepare.

**If you prefer to work out fasted, stay hydrated.** Sip water or an electrolyte drink throughout your workout to sustain energy and prevent dehydration. Fasted workouts work well for lower-intensity or early morning sessions.

**If you eat before your workout, 30 to 90 minutes before-hand, consume a mix of protein and carbs,** something light and easy to digest, such as Greek yogurt with fruit or a protein shake with a banana. Adjust the timing based on how you feel.

## Intra-Workout: Sustaining Energy for Long Rucks

For regular rucks under an hour, plain water should keep you hydrated. Longer or more intense workouts, such as in the 10K or 25K training plans, require additional energy and electrolyte support, especially in hot or humid climates.

Finding the right mix of nutrients and timing takes experimentation. Some endurance athletes start their intra-workout fueling too late. Falling behind can lead to poor performance or the feeling of "hitting a wall," which can prove difficult to overcome mid-session. To avoid this, stay on schedule with your hydration and nutrition during extended rucks, especially as you enter the final weeks of a 10K or 25K training plan. Practice intra-workout fueling strategies during training rucks so you have a solid plan come race day.

Consider these guidelines to help you stay fueled during rucks lasting more than 60 or 90 minutes:

**Hydration:** Drink 16 to 24 ounces per hour. Adjust your intake based on your sweat rate, workout intensity, and weather conditions. Pre-filling your water bottles helps track your intake and pace accordingly.

**Electrolytes and sodium:** Fluids alone aren't enough. Electrolyte powders or drinks with sodium help prevent cramps and dehydration. Replace sodium losses with 250 to 500 mg per hour, especially if you sweat a lot. For optimal hydration, look for an electrolyte supplement with at least 300 mg of sodium per serving. Nuun, LMNT, Liquid I.V., and similar products fit the bill. Otherwise, save money and simply add a pinch of salt to your water bottle.

**Carbs:** Consume 30 to 50 grams of carbohydrates per hour. Quick options include energy gels or chews, sports drinks with carbs, or portable snacks such as dried fruit, granola bars, or graham crackers. This is the perfect time to put some of your favorite candy or "fast" carbs to good use.

As you approach the end of your workout, start thinking about recovery. Rehydrating and replenishing glycogen stores will help your body bounce back stronger for the next session.

## *Post-Workout: Replenishing for the Next Session*

Recovery starts the moment your workout ends. It's not just about bouncing back from a tough session; it's about setting yourself up for the next one. When you give your body what it needs to replenish and repair itself, your hard work won't go to waste.

A well-rounded post-workout meal or snack can make all the difference. Include a mixture of carbs and high-quality protein. A whey protein shake blended with fruit makes a convenient option. Grilled chicken or tofu with quinoa and roasted vegetables or a turkey sandwich with whole-grain bread offers balance and variety.

For intermediate and heavy rucks or workouts lasting more than one to two hours, consider these fueling recommendations.

| Dietary Considerations | Pre-workout | Intra-workout | Post-workout |
|---|---|---|---|
| General | Cottage cheese with pineapple and hemp hearts<br><br>Scrambled eggs on avocado toast<br><br>Bagel with cream cheese and smoked salmon | Electrolyte drink and a banana<br><br>Trail mix<br><br>Peanut butter and jelly sandwich | Grilled chicken pita with veggies and hummus<br><br>Turkey and cheese wrap with green salad<br><br>Salmon with rice and asparagus |
| Gluten-free | Oatmeal with almond butter and whey protein<br><br>Scrambled eggs with sweet potato hash<br><br>Greek yogurt with gluten-free granola and berries | Dried mango and almonds<br><br>Gluten-free granola bar<br><br>Coconut water with dates and nuts | Steak fajita with corn tortillas<br><br>Salmon with sweet potatoes and greens<br><br>Sausage and lentil soup with veggies |
| Dairy-free | Smoothie (banana, collagen powder, almond milk)<br><br>Chia pudding with berries and hemp seeds<br><br>Egg, avocado, and ham sandwich | Coconut water with dried fruit and nuts<br><br>Electrolyte drink and an apple or a banana<br><br>Graham crackers with nut butter | Poké bowl with avocado and cucumber<br><br>Chicken and veggie stir-fry with rice<br><br>Tuna salad with chickpeas, mixed greens, and tahini dressing |

| Dietary Considerations | Pre-workout | Intra-workout | Post-workout |
|---|---|---|---|
| Vegetarian/ Vegan | Chia pudding with coconut milk and cherries<br><br>Peanut butter toast with banana slices<br><br>Overnight oats with pea protein powder | Trail mix and applesauce packet<br><br>Coconut water with banana chips and walnuts<br><br>Sports drink and pretzel sticks | Tofu or tempeh stir-fry with rice and broccoli<br><br>Lentil soup with quinoa<br><br>Black bean tacos with avocado and salsa |
| Low-carb/ Keto | Scrambled eggs with avocado and cheese<br><br>Whole-milk Greek yogurt with nuts and seeds<br><br>BLT sandwich on keto bread | Electrolyte drink, nuts, and cheese crisps<br><br>Beef jerky or pork rinds<br><br>Peanut or almond butter packet | Grass-fed beef with cauliflower mash and Brussels sprouts<br><br>Grilled shrimp and vegetable skewers<br><br>Chicken thighs with sautéed mushrooms and zucchini |
| Allergen-friendly<br><br>(no nuts, eggs, fish/ shellfish, dairy, soy, gluten) | Quinoa porridge with berries and pumpkin seeds<br><br>Banana, coconut milk, and protein powder smoothie<br><br>Turkey roll-ups with cucumber slices and hummus | Apple slices with sunflower seed butter<br><br>Dried coconut and raisins<br><br>Rice cakes with honey and banana slices | Lettuce-wrapped bison burger with roasted sweet potato fries<br><br>Chicken and quinoa bowl with roasted vegetables<br><br>Venison stew with vegetables |

▶ ▶ ▶

Sometimes recovery requires more than food. A handful of supplements can help you perform better and recover faster:

**Creatine:** This safe, affordable, well-studied supplement supports workout performance, strength gains, and even brain health. Take 5 grams of creatine monohydrate daily, even on rest days, to enhance performance and aid recovery.[33]

**Magnesium:** This powerhouse mineral helps with hundreds of body processes: energy production, insulin signaling, muscle repair, sleep, and more. It comes in different forms with varying absorption. Aim for at least 300 mg of elemental magnesium per day.[38]

**Vitamin D:** Essential for bone health, immunity, insulin, and muscle function, this micronutrient can enhance recovery and overall performance. Have your level tested regularly and know that, like many biomarkers, "normal" does not mean "optimal." For vitamin $D_3$, the RDA runs between 600 and 800 IU per day. Some experts recommend up to 1,500 or 2,000 IU daily.[39] These numbers represent maintenance doses, so work with your healthcare provider to correct any known deficiency.

**Whey protein:** Meeting your protein needs through food alone can prove challenging. Whey protein offers a high-quality, cost-effective way to supply your body with the necessary amino acids for muscle preservation and repair.

Recovery doesn't end with fluids, food, and vitamins. Sleep plays a critical role, too. Prioritize seven to nine hours of quality sleep per night to give your body time to rejuvenate and prepare for the next workout. Combine consistent sleep, a well-balanced diet, and the three stages of fueling to create a strong foundation for performance and progress.

## REMEMBER

► Don't let what you eat dictate how you move. Movement isn't punishment for what you ate. Eating and exercise are forms of self-respect.

► If you want to lose weight, focus on fat loss rather than weight loss. Remember that eating fat doesn't make you fat. Eating excess calories does, but not all calories are created equal.

► Eating for blood sugar balance can help you tackle emotional eating, overcome energy crashes, and avoid stubborn cravings, ultimately helping you lose and maintain weight while optimizing metabolic health.

► Protein is a daily nonnegotiable, because we can't store it like other macronutrients. Calculate your protein target based on your fitness goals and distribute your intake throughout the day.

► Eat more slow carbs and fewer fast carbs. Consider using a continuous glucose monitor to assess your personal tolerance for carbohydrates.

► Test and fine-tune your pre-, intra-, and post-workout nutrition plan for long rucks and other strenuous workouts. If you're signed up for an event, race day is not the time to experiment with new fueling strategies.

# 6

## Embrace the Ruck

Words may inspire,
but only action creates change.

—SIMON SINEK,
AUTHOR

n today's world, we've become experts at avoiding discomfort: 24/7 climate control, same-day delivery, memory foam every-thing, and food at our fingertips. We dodge anything that is even remotely unpleasant, especially exercise. We binge-watch our favorite TV series and listen to podcasts to distract ourselves while we "close rings" and meet the minimum activity require-ments for the day. But here's the kicker: A bit of physical distress, such as a challenging ruck, goes a long way. When you proactively seek discomfort, you build toughness, rewire your brain to handle stress better, and achieve a sense of accomplishment. Discomfort, it turns out, is the secret sauce for growth.

# HABITS > GOALS

To begin a self-improvement journey, most people start by setting a goal. But let's talk about why habits, not goals, are the real agents for creating lasting change.

Goals are great to get going. They give you a target, a reason to get started. But what happens after you reach your goal? If you don't have solid habits, you risk drifting backward and losing your progress—or worse, returning to square one, as often happens with people who set unrealistic weight loss goals. Prioritizing habits over goals changes the game. Habits keep you grounded and consistent while goals are more fleeting.

Overcoming bad habits or initiating good ones involves plenty of discomfort. Changing habits disrupts your routine. It feels uncomfortable at first—just like your first few rucks. But over time, your body adapts, your mind toughens, and it feels easier. The more you practice, the more automatic your habits become. Practice makes progress. Consider these tips to help you start strong and stay consistent.

**Use a habit tracker.** Whether it's an app or a notebook, keeping tabs on progress can be motivating, especially if you're like me and love checking boxes. You can find a free printable habit tracker on my website (kaylagirgenrd.com/free-habit-tracker-printable).

**Set up your environment for success.** Make good habits easy to maintain. Keep your rucksack packed and by the door. Move unhealthy foods out of sight and meal-prep healthy snacks to grab and go. Remove any friction between you and the habits you want to build.

**Leverage accountability.** Share your goals with a friend, post your progress on social media, or hire a coach. Accountability is a powerful tool for follow-through. If you're a people pleaser, it's an exceptional method: You succeed because you don't want to let others down.

**Stack good habits.** In the book *Atomic Habits,* James Clear explains how one of the simplest ways to start a new habit is to pair it with an existing one. Embedded habits act as triggers for new ones. For example, turning on the coffee pot in the morning can remind you to stretch for five minutes.

However strong your habits, patterns always come with the risk of disruption. Life's interruptions, planned and unplanned, can happen for better or worse. For example, you might press pause on a habit for a family vacation or to keep up with work obligations, making it tempting to revert to comfort or unhealthy vices. Recognizing this risk gives you the opportunity to develop strategies to bounce back quickly. Preparedness and resilience can make all the difference.

# ELIMINATE EXCUSES BY MAKING HABIT CHANGE EASY

Sticking with a new habit shouldn't feel like a monumental task. If you bite off more than you can chew, you might procrastinate or conjure up excuses before you even get going. Easy can seem bad or lazy, but in this case, it's the opposite. Easy is good when you start something new. Easy gets you going, and that's the hardest part.

Overplanning and procrastination, on the other hand, can prevent you from taking action. When you wait for life to slow down or promise to begin tomorrow, Monday, next month, or January, you waste time waiting for the right time. What started simply as a goal to "work out" spirals into a whirlwind of unrealistic expectations and analysis paralysis. You stop before you even start.

With rucking, it's easy *and* good to start small. A 10-minute walk with a light pack can boost your mood, encouraging you to do it again. Opting for easy makes it more likely you'll build momentum and motivation. Because rucking can be as simple as walking, it has no learning curve. You don't have to stare at a treadmill console or navigate a crowded gym. Just load your pack, put on some sturdy shoes, and head outside.

Making exercise easy removes excuses, so you literally can get a move on. Easy may not seem sexy or exciting, but it's effective. Easy is practical and attainable. Meet yourself where you are and aim to improve incrementally. Forget all-or-nothing thinking and embrace the snowball effect of small, compounding change. Every ruck doesn't have to be an epic adventure, so the next time you feel like skipping a workout, just grab your pack and go. It's that easy.

# MANAGING TIME AND ENERGY FOR MAXIMUM GAINS

It's equally important to manage your energy efficiently. It helps to consider which habits you can maintain on your worst days. For example, you won't wake up feeling 100 percent every single day. Some days, you might feel like you're running on fumes. Give yourself some grace. If you have only half a tank and you give all 50 percent that day, you've given it your all, and that's a win. Showing up, even when you're not at your best, builds consistency and character. Your performance on bad days is often what matters most.

Many people struggle with consistency because they aim for perfection. The second they fall short of perfect, they quit. To avoid giving up, implement this good-better-best system to tier your expectations, which allows for day-to-day flexibility while still practicing persistence.

**Good:** The baseline you can achieve even on tough days (a walk around the block)

**Better:** A realistic target for an average day (5,000 steps)

**Best:** A stretch goal for when you feel motivated and energized (10,000 steps)

Tiering your goals keeps you moving forward and prevents you from falling into an all-or-nothing mindset. Some days are just "good," and that's OK as long as you stay consistent. Learning how to manage your energy and distractions, especially in the face of discomfort and bad days, matters most for long-term success.

But that means deciding what matters and ensuring your actions follow suit. Health, family, financial security, whatever we deem important can take a back seat to life's more immediate demands. For example, if "being healthy" tops your list, yet you skip a workout to binge Netflix, a lack of time isn't the issue; it's a *perceived* lack of time. How you spend your time isn't aligning with your goals, which makes it a *priority* problem, not a time problem.

If "I don't have time" tops your list of excuses for skipping workouts, rucking can work for you. It fits effortlessly into your day. You don't need to block an entire hour or drive to the gym. Grab a backpack, add some weight, and head out the door. You can ruck on your lunch break, as you're shopping for groceries, or while walking the dog. It can work around your life, not the other way around. And every step counts, making it easy to stay active no matter how packed your schedule.

Still skeptical? Think of exercise as time *invested*, not time spent. When you prioritize fitness, you probably perform better in all aspects of life. Movement breeds movement—in many ways.

When you make time to work out, you're more likely to make healthier food choices, connect with those you love, and meet deadlines on time.

If you still feel overwhelmed, consider the Four Burners Theory. In a *New Yorker* article, David Sedaris described life as a stove with four burners, one each for health, family, friends, and work. To be successful, you have to shut off one burner. To be extraordinarily successful, you have to shut off two.[40] It's a simple, yet incredibly effective way to pinpoint and manage your priorities. You decide what goes on the back burner(s).

Unlike many other forms of exercise, rucking allows you to tackle two burners at once. If health and family top your list, plan a family ruck. If friends and health matter most, ruck with a friend rather than catching up at a bar. If work ranks highest, ruck on your lunch break to clear your head and generate fresh ideas. Whatever's on your stove right now, your priorities will evolve and change. You'll have to turn burners up and down, on and off, throughout the different seasons of life. Rucking lets you double dip, so your health stays on the front burner, no matter what else is cooking.

# TRACKING PROGRESS FOR SUSTAINABLE SUCCESS

Monitoring your efforts over time not only creates a record of your success but also generates momentum. Tracking your progress provides data that you can use to your advantage. Whether logging mileage or gradually increasing ruck weight, measuring these improvements provides a confidence boost along with valuable insights into your overall performance. It also holds you accountable. It's harder to skip a workout or go easy on a ruck when you have a daily mileage goal staring back at you. Data helps you identify what's working and what's not so you can tweak your approach for optimal results.

For tracking progress, there's no one-size-fits-all approach. Experiment to find what gels best with your personality and training objectives. For instance, if you're training for a race, you might prefer a structured system with detailed mileage and pace logs. If you want to drop body fat, progress photos or a body composition analysis might work for you. Find a method that's motivating and feels manageable, not like a chore. Otherwise, you won't follow through with it. Consider these options:

**Fitness trackers:** Wearable devices or smartphone apps log mileage, heart rate, and calories burned. Many provide trends, helping you monitor improvements over time.

**Special apps:** RuckWell and other free apps record specific metrics, such as "ruck work" and "ruck power," giving detailed data from each training session.

**Habit trackers:** Hang a paper tracker or your *Ruck Fit* training plan somewhere prominent and cross off workouts. Seeing the checkmarks add up is incredibly satisfying.

**Journals:** For a more detailed approach, log workouts in a training journal. This method works especially well for strength training, helping you keep tabs on how much weight you lifted and set goals for future sessions. Use a notebook or purchase a fitness journal online.

**Photos or videos:** Snap a picture or take video during your ruck or workout sessions. Comparing side-by-side evidence of your progress over weeks or months can be rewarding, especially for physical changes or skill development.

Start small. Begin with one data point to monitor your progress: time, distance, weight, or completion of a session. Once the habit is more established, layer in more details to create a clearer picture of your progress. Concrete data remove ambiguity about whether you're improving. If you're not progressing as fast as you'd like, identify trends and adjust your approach to deliver better results. Looking back over weeks or months, you'll see how far you've come. The data doesn't lie.

## STAYING MOTIVATED WHEN THE GOING GETS TOUGH

No matter how hard you work, progress will feel slow some days. Life gets busy, and motivation ebbs and flows. Setbacks are inevitable and normal. That's why it's so important to have strategies in place to help you bounce back when challenges arise. When your motivation wavers, use these tips to stay on track and maintain momentum:

**Revisit your "why."** Remind yourself of the reason you started. Reconnecting with your purpose can reignite your motivation. Write down your goals and keep them visible as a daily reminder of what you're working toward.

**Focus on small wins.** When progress feels slow, look back at the data you collected or compare visuals to remind yourself how far you've come. Recognizing even the littlest of victories keeps you moving forward. Slow progress is still progress.

**Adjust, don't abandon.** Whatever you do, don't quit. If life throws you a curveball, modify your plan instead of giving up. Adaptability is one of the most valuable skills you can cultivate to stay on course and overcome obstacles.

**Lean on support.** Share your goals with a friend, join a ruck club, or work with a coach who can help you troubleshoot setbacks. Ask family for help with household chores and accept that their ways might differ from yours. You can't do it all or be everything to everyone. Know your limits and recruit help as needed. Asking for help is a sign of strength, not weakness.

**Move on.** Everyone has off days. Don't dwell on a missed workout or a lousy training session. Acknowledge that slipups happen. Treat them as learning opportunities, focus on what you can do differently next time, and keep moving forward.

Motivation isn't always consistent, but your commitment can be. By having a contingency plan and focusing on the bigger picture, you'll be able to overcome challenges and stay on track. The road to success isn't always smooth, but it's always worth it.

## REMEMBER

▶ Goals get you started, but habits keep you going. Once you reach a goal, it's your habits that sustain your success.

▶ Accept easy. Start small and enjoy the benefits of compounding change.

▶ Track your progress to assess improvements and maintain motivation.

▶ Reframe inevitable setbacks as learning opportunities for next time. Adapt and adjust, but don't quit.

# Conclusion

The finish line is just
the beginning of a whole new race.

—UNKNOWN

R ucking dates back thousands of years, but its modern appeal lies in its accessibility and effectiveness. This cornerstone of military training has evolved into a mainstream, recreational activity, and for good reason. It builds muscle, strengthens bones, and boosts metabolic health. It can help ward off chronic illness, improve fitness, and fortify overall quality of life—all that with just a backpack and a little weight. Sometimes the most straightforward solutions prove most effective.

But the real magic of rucking goes beyond the physical. It gets you out of your head and into the outdoors; it's nature's ultimate mood booster. It helps relieve stress, foster mindfulness and resilience, and, if you like, cultivate meaningful connections with others. Whether you're strolling through your neighborhood or exploring a scenic trail, rucking invites you to move with purpose and presence.

It's simple, therapeutic, and free. It's just an exercise, but it can become a way of life. Your rucksack can turn into the most versatile, reliable gym buddy you'll ever have. Toss it on while mowing the lawn, walking the dog, or running errands. Multitask your workout, maximize your time, and ruck anytime, anywhere, with anyone. Endlessly adaptable, rucking fits into your life, not the other way around.

By now, I hope you feel inspired to give rucking a try. If you haven't tried it yet, you owe it to yourself to experience the transformative benefits of walking with weight. One of the biggest mistakes you can make is not doing it. Don't overthink it. Just grab your ruck and go.

So what are you waiting for? You don't need a perfect plan, a membership to anything, or even the "right" gear. All you need is a willingness to start—right here, right now, with what you have. So grab yourself a backpack, throw in some weight, and go for a walk. The next step is yours.

# Acknowledgments

If you surround yourself with love
and the right people, anything is possible.

—ADAM GREEN,
ACTOR AND SCREENWRITER

My deepest gratitude goes to Dalyn Miller and the incredible team at Torsk Media, including Alanya Telerski. Your steadfast support, humor, and endless wisdom proved invaluable as I navigated the uncharted territory of writing my first book. Thank you for having faith in me. Without you, this journey wouldn't have been possible.

To James Jayo, Emma Peters, and the editorial team at Countryman Press: From the very beginning, I knew this book was in the right hands. Thank you for taking a chance on me and recognizing the potential of *Ruck Fit*. Your shared vision and guidance helped shape this book. Bravo to Chrissy Kurpeski for the brilliant book design. Your creativity truly brought the pages to life, and I couldn't be happier with the final result. I'm beyond thankful to the entire team at Countryman Press—editors, proofreaders, designers, marketers, and everyone involved in sales. Your work, seen and unseen, ensured that this book came to life and reached readers ready to transform their lives. Each of you played an essential role in making this project a reality, and I am honored to have had your expertise and dedication behind it.

Erika Hansen, thank you for your incredible work behind the camera. Your enthusiasm for this project was contagious, and you made the photoshoot feel easy and comfortable. I can't say thank you enough for that! You delivered stunning images on a tight deadline with the attention to detail that was needed to make the entire process seamless and professional.

To the North Star Ruck Club: Your camaraderie and our group rucks served as a lifeline during the writing process. Each mile rucked together reminded me why I was writing this book—to inspire, to connect, and to help others find strength through movement. You all kept me grounded and centered, and I'm truly appreciative of the role you played.

To my high school English teachers Mr. Makela and Mrs. Menden: Thank you for seeing potential in a teenager who didn't understand the value of good writing. Your thoughtful guidance and gentle nudges to keep improving laid the foundation for the writer I am today. I appreciate you more than words can express.

To my friends, family, followers, and clients: Your unwavering encouragement and patience have meant the world to me. Thank you for your endless support and grace as I declined countless outings to meet deadlines. To my husband, Jeremy, the ultimate teammate and cheerleader, you have been my rock throughout this journey. Your persistent accountability kept me on course, and your willingness to take on extra responsibilities allowed me to pour my all into this project. You were the protector of my time, energy, and sanity. Thank you for your selflessness and for always doing the dishes so I didn't have to.

To everyone involved in making this book—and to everyone reading it—this is as much yours as it is mine, and I'm forever grateful.

# Resources

## APPS

AllTrails (www.alltrails.com)
RuckWell (ruckwell.com)
Strava (www.strava.com)
Carb Manager (www.carbmanager.com)
Cronometer (cronometer.com)
Lose It! (www.loseit.com)

## WEBSITES

GORUCK: Rucking Calorie Calculator: www.goruck.com/pages/
    rucking-calorie-calculator
Ruck for Miles: Rucking Calorie Calculator: www.ruckformiles
    .com/guides/calories-burned-rucking-calculator
*Outside*: The Ultimate Backpacking Calorie Estimator: www
    .outsideonline.com/outdoor-adventure/hiking-and
    -backpacking/ultimate-backpacking-calorie-estimator
iPB: Protein Calculator: www.internationalproteinboard.org/
    post/how-much-protein-is-right-for-me

Stay up-to-date with my favorite resources, snacks, and supplements by signing up for my weekly email newsletter at www
.wintheweek.gr8.com. Visit my website for more free resources:
www.kaylagirgenrd.com.

# Recommended Reading

Today a reader, tomorrow a leader.

—MARGARET FULLER

Over the years, certain books have shaped my views on physical and mental health, sparking meaningful change in my life, health, and work, as well as in the lives of my clients. The following books on health, nutrition, and mindset encouraged me to think differently, transformed my practice, and provided invaluable tools and strategies I still use today. I hope you find them as inspiring and helpful as I did.

## HABITS AND GOALS

*Atomic Habits: An Easy & Proven Way to Build Good Habits & Break Bad Ones* by James Clear
Small, consistent actions can compound into remarkable results, helping you build good habits and break bad ones. If you haven't picked up this bestseller yet, consider this your nudge to start.

*Better Than Before: What I Learned about Making and Breaking Habits—To Sleep More, Quit Sugar, Procrastinate Less, and Generally Build a Happier Life* by Gretchen Rubin
Learn which of the Four Tendencies suits you best and discover a framework that leverages your strengths to make healthy habits stick.

*Finish: Give Yourself the Gift of Done* by Jon Acuff
With a refreshing mix of humor and practical wisdom, Acuff offers strategies to set realistic goals so you can overcome perfectionism, get out of your own way, and stay motivated all the way to the finish line.

# HEALTH AND NUTRITION

*Glucose Revolution: The Life-Changing Power of Balancing Your Blood Sugar* by Jessie Inchauspé
Packed with practical tips and insights, this book is an excellent introduction to the ins and outs of blood sugar management, including food sources prone to creating glucose spikes and actionable strategies to help blunt them.

*In Defense of Food: An Eater's Manifesto* by Michael Pollan
In this inspiring guide to rediscovering the joy of eating and cooking, Pollan simplifies the complexity of modern diets with his iconic mantra: "Eat food. Not too much. Mostly plants."

*The Obesity Code: Unlocking the Secrets of Weight Loss* by Jason Fung, MD
Dr. Fung challenges conventional advice by presenting obesity as a hormonal imbalance involving insulin, rather than just a caloric surplus, suggesting intermittent fasting, dietary adjustments, and

other strategies to regulate insulin levels, aiming for sustainable weight loss and improved health.

*Outlive: The Science & Art of Longevity* by Peter Attia, MD
With a critical look at the gaps in modern healthcare, Dr. Attia shares actionable strategies for preventative health that emphasize physical, mental, and emotional well-being.

*Sacred Cow: The Case for (Better) Meat: Why Well-Raised Meat Is Good for You and Good for the Planet* by Diana Rodgers, RD
In this thought-provoking exploration of the role of meat in our diets, health, and the environment, Rodgers makes a compelling case for sustainable and regenerative agriculture, offering a nuanced perspective on eating better for our bodies and the planet.

# LIFESTYLE AND MINDSET

*The Comfort Crisis: Embrace Discomfort to Reclaim Your Wild, Happy, Healthy Self* by Michael Easter
Through engaging stories and research, Easter explores how pushing limits can transform mental and physical health. This book is how I first discovered rucking.

*The Mountain Is You: Transforming Self-Sabotage into Self-Mastery* by Brianna Wiest
Exploring the root causes of self-sabotage, Wiest offers insights and actionable strategies for overcoming the internal obstacles that hold you back.

*The War of Art: Break Through the Blocks and Win Your Inner Creative Battles* by Steven Pressfield
With sharp insights and practical advice, Pressfield exposes the

barriers that hold us back from pursuing our passions and achieving our goals. After reading this book, my husband quit his job to pursue his own business; it's that powerful.

*When Food Is Comfort: Nurture Yourself Mindfully, Rewire Your Brain, and End Emotional Eating* by Julie M. Simon
Simon explores the roots of food-related coping mechanisms, especially those formed in childhood, and provides tools to rewire your brain and nurture yourself in healthier ways that don't involve food.

*Winning: The Unforgiving Race to Greatness* by Tim S. Grover
Drawing from his experience training Michael Jordan, Kobe Bryant, and other elite athletes, Grover presents 13 principles that define the path to victory, emphasizing the necessity of unwavering commitment, mental toughness, and embracing discomfort.

# Notes

1. Edwards, T., and Ward, S. (2022). "Rucking: A Low-Impact, High Cardio Exercise Option." *Healthline.*
2. Taylor, N. A., Peoples, G. E., and Petersen, S. R. (2016). "Load Carriage, Human Performance, and Employment Standards." *Applied Physiology, Nutrition, and Metabolism* 41, no. 6 (Suppl 2): S131–S147.
3. Barrell, A. (2023). "What Happens to the Body after Sitting Down for Too Long?" *Medical News Today.*
4. WHO Media Team. (2024). "Nearly 1.8 Billion Adults at Risk of Disease from Not Doing Enough Physical Activity." World Health Organization.
5. Taylor, N. A., et al. (2016). "Load Carriage, Human Performance." *Applied Physiology, Nutrition, and Metabolism* 41, no. 6 (Suppl. 2): S131–S147.
6. Siemandel, J. (2021). "Guardsmen Earn Norwegian Foot March Badge during Joint Event." National Guard.
7. Human Foods Program. (2018). "Guidance for Industry: Guide for Developing and Using Data Bases for Nutrition Labeling." Food and Drug Administration.
8. Alcohol and Drug Foundation. (2023). "What Is Hangxiety?" ADF Insights.
9. Khubchandani, J., Price, J., Sharma, S., Wiblishhauser, M., and Webb, F. (2022). "COVID-19 Pandemic and Weight Gain in American Adults: A Nationwide Population-Based Study." *Diabetes & Metabolic Syndrome* 16, no. 1: 102392.
10. Angus, C., Buckley, C., Tilstra, A. M., and Dowd, J. B. (2023). "Increases in 'Deaths of Despair' during the COVID-19 Pandemic in the United States and the United Kingdom." *Public Health* 218: 92–96.
11. Vogel, S. (2023). "Healthcare Worker Exodus Continued through 2022, New Data Shows." Healthcare Dive.
12. EPA. (2024.) "Indoor Air Quality." US Environmental Protection Agency Report on the Environment.
13. GilPress. (2023). "Average Screen Time Statistics." What's the Big Data.
14. Office of the Surgeon General. (2023). "Our Epidemic of Loneliness and Isolation." US Department of Health and Human Services.

15. Thyfault, J. P., and Bergouignan, A. (2020). "Exercise and Metabolic Health: Beyond Skeletal Muscle." *Diabetologia* 63, no. 8: 1464–74.
16. Kim, G., and Kim, J. H. (2020). "Impact of Skeletal Muscle Mass on Metabolic Health." *Endocrinology and Metabolism* 35, no. 1: 1–6.
17. Edemekong, P. F., Bomgaars, D. L., Sukumaran, S., and Schoo, C. (2025). "Activities of Daily Living." In *StatPearls*. StatPearls Publishing.
18. McCall, P. (2023). "The Surprising Benefits of Rucking (and Why Your Clients Might Love It)." *Certified Magazine*. May 2023.
19. Sherriff, A. "Rucking Calorie Calculator—How Many Calories Are Burned Rucking?" Ruck for Miles.
20. Drain, J. R., Aisbett, B., Lewis, M., and Billing, D. C. (2017). "The Pandolf Equation Under-Predicts the Metabolic Rate of Contemporary Military Load Carriage. *Journal of Science and Medicine in Sport* 20, no. 4: S104–S108.
21. Chen, L. R., Hou, P. H., and Chen, K. H. (2019). "Nutritional Support and Physical Modalities for People with Osteoporosis: Current Opinion." *Nutrients* 11, no. 12: 2848.
22. Webb, C. E., Rossignac-Milon, M., and Higgins, E. T. (2017). "Stepping Forward Together: Could Walking Facilitate Interpersonal Conflict Resolution?" *The American Psychologist* 72, no. 4: 374–85.
23. Barton, J., Bragg, R., Wood, C., and Pretty, J. (2016). *Green Exercise: Linking Nature, Health and Well-Being* (1st ed.). Routledge.
24. Raichlen, D. A., and Lieberman, D. E. (2022). "The Evolution of Human Step Counts and Its Association with the Risk of Chronic Disease." *Current Biology* 32, no. 21: R1206–R1214.
25. Thyfault, J. P., and Bergouignan, A. (2020). "Exercise and Metabolic Health: Beyond Skeletal Muscle." *Diabetologia* 63, no. 8: 1464–74.
26. Genitrini, M., Dotti, F., Bianca, E., and Ferri, A. (2022). "Impact of Backpacks on Ergonomics: Biomechanical and Physiological Effects: A Narrative Review." *International Journal of Environmental Research and Public Health* 19, no. 11: 6737.
27. Orr, R., Pope, R., Lopes, T. J. A., Leyk, D., Blacker, S., Bustillo-Aguirre, B. S., and Knapik, J. J. (2021). "Soldier Load Carriage, Injuries, Rehabilitation and Physical Conditioning: An International Approach." *International Journal of Environmental Research and Public Health* 18, no. 8: 4010.
28. Genitrini, M., et al. "Impact of Backpacks on Ergonomics: Biomechanical and Physiological Effects. A Narrative Review." *International Journal of Environmental Research and Public Health* 19, no. 11: 6737.
29. Marshall, M. (2022). "Mobility." Harvard Health Publishing, Harvard Medical School.

30. Kansas State University. "Food Product Development." (2024). Kansas Value Added Foods Lab.

31. Raichle, M. E, and Gusnard, D.A. (2002). "Appraising the Brain's Energy Budget." *Proceedings of the National Academy of Sciences* 99, no.: 10237–239.

32. National Academies of Sciences, Engineering, and Medicine. (2023). "Factors Affecting Energy Expenditure and Requirements." In *Dietary Reference Intakes for Energy.* The National Academies Press.

33. Gropper, S., and Smith, J. (2013). *Advanced Nutrition and Human Metabolism* (6th edition). Cengage Learning.

34. International Protein Board. "How Much Protein Is Right For Me?" www .internationalproteinboard.org/post/how-much-protein-is-right-for-me.

35. Layman D. K. (2024). "Impacts of Protein Quantity and Distribution on Body Composition." *Frontiers in Nutrition* 11: 1388986.

36. Chang, C. Y., Ke, D. S., and Chen, J. Y. (2009). "Essential Fatty Acids and Human Brain." *Acta Neurologica Taiwanica* 18, no. 4: 231–41.

37. Nesti, L., Mengozzi, A., and Tricò, D. (2019). "Impact of Nutrient Type and Sequence on Glucose Tolerance: Physiological Insights and Therapeutic Implications." *Frontiers in Endocrinology* 10: 144.

38. Dean, C. (2017). *The Magnesium Miracle* (Second Edition). Ballantine Books.

39. Eckelkamp, S. (2023). "Do You Get Enough Vitamin D? Here's How It Benefits Metabolic Health." *Levels* (blog).

40. Sedaris, David. (2009). "Laugh, Kookaburra." *The New Yorker.* August 24, 2009.

# Index

# About the Author

**Kayla Girgen, CPT, RD, LD** is a certified personal trainer and a registered and licensed dietitian. She completed her supervised practice at the Mayo Clinic in Rochester, Minnesota. Specializing in weight management and habit change, Kayla debunks fitness and nutrition myths and helps people optimize their metabolic health. Her work has appeared in the pages of *Men's Health, Parade, Forbes, Health, Insider, Livestrong,* and other media outlets. She lives in Minnesota with her husband, Jeremy.